CARDIOFITNESS
Can Save Your Life __

CARDIOFITNESS
Can Save Your Life __

Forrest Blanding

BASCOM HILL
PUBLISHING GROUP

Bascom Hill Publishing Group
212 3rd Avenue North, Suite 570
Minneapolis, MN 55401
612.455.2293
www.bascomhillpublishing.com

ISBN - 978-1-935098-04-1
ISBN - 1-935098-04-7
LCCN - 2008935433

Book sales for North America and international:
Itasca Books, 3501 Highway 100 South, Suite 220
Minneapolis, MN 55416
Phone: 952.345.4488 (toll free 1.800.901.3480)
Fax: 952.920.0541; email to orders@itascabooks.com

Cover Design by Paul Shively
Typeset by Tiffany Laschinger

Printed in the United States of America

BASCOM HILL
PUBLISHING GROUP

From a Review of this book by
Dr. Kenneth H. Cooper, M.D., M.P.H

"Your book is excellent, has a lot of potential"

and

"There is a much needed audience for books of this type who could benefit immeasurably"

Dr Cooper is well known throughout the world as the "Father of Aerobic Exercise" His landmark book "Aerobics" in 1968 motivated millions to start doing proper aerobic exercise. He founded the famous Cooper Aerobics Center in Dallas in 1970.

He also founded the Cooper Institute for Aerobics Research, a non-profit organization that has produced the key research on exercise and health, and the Cooper Institute that provides today's most up-to-date preventative medicine.

Dr Cooper has authored about twenty books on exercise and other health related subjects and is widely regarded as the top world authority on exercise... .

PROLOGUE

The world of health is obsessed with EXERCISE. You read it in the paper. You see it in every magazine about health. You read about it in books. EXERCISE is claimed to help nearly every physical, emotional, sexual or other problem we have. The advice tiresomely says, "Do your Exercise."

But key questions remain: What exercise? How much exercise? We hear again and again the advice to walk 30 minutes each or most days. This is a lot of our free time. Will this cure all those problems caused by lack of exercise? Eighty percent of men and women doing exercise claim that they do this for their health. A majority say that they walk. Yet today's research shows that millions are now wasting vast amounts of time pursuing trivial health benefits by incorrectly walking 30 minutes every day. Or even walking 60 minutes every day. In fact, most people that exercise have little idea about the health value of what they are doing.

I will show here how most can gain far more for their health from lesser times of exercise. Those that do not exercise have little idea of the damage this can be causing to their health and life.

Before the mid-1990's we were told to exercise to some percentage of maximum heart rate. This led to millions of people running, swimming and doing aerobics. Is that 'percentage of maximum heart rate' for exercise now passé? Is high-level exercise really necessary? How about that popular bodybuilding. Will this really make us healthier?

The experts now tell us to exercise, as a minimum, either 'moderately' five days a week for 30 minutes or 'vigorously' three days a week for 20 minutes. This is better than their previous hopelessly inadequate advice. But you deserve a more scientific program than this. You deserve not just a more solidly-based minimum program but options for much more healthful programs. You deserve to know how to develop real benefits from your exercise, effectively and efficiently, from the exercises you prefer to do.

Correct exercise is vastly more important to our health and future than has been realized. The key is cardiofitness. What is called 'exercise' reduces a risk of a heart attack of 1.5 to 2 times. Cardiofitness can reduce risk at least 5 to 10 times. What is called 'exercise' may reduce risk of some cancers somewhat. Cardiofitness can identify a 3 to 4 times lower risks of breast, colon, prostrate and nearly all other causes of cancer. Cardiofitness substantially reduces risk of diabetes, Alzheimer's, lung disease, macular degeneration and other major disease. I show that poor cardiofitness can be more harmful to our health than cholesterol, blood pressure, or even smoking cigarettes.

Cardiofitness (also called cardiorespitory fitness, cardiovascular fitness and physical fitness) is not new. It was introduced to the public by Dr. Kenneth Cooper in 1968 in his best-selling book Aerobics. My previous book The Pulse Point Plan, (Random House 1982) provided a first scientific verification of its importance. Yet incredibly, recognition of cardiofitness has been dying for more than a dozen years. We have a new generation of supposed exercise experts that seem to know little about it. We now have 'official' recommendations that fail to even mention it.

This book shows for the first time, from more than twenty years of scientific analysis, how exercise benefits health. A new theory from this analysis deserves to be called revolutionary because it upsets so many wrong ideas about how exercise benefits us. This new Heart Theory of Exercise and Cardiofitness shows that 85% of the exercise benefits to our health develop from the cardiofitness it produces. Cardiofitness is a measurable physical condition of our heart and its accompanying cardiovascular muscle that can be improved only by aerobic exercise. Exercise that does not contribute to cardiofitness – and this is much of what many now do – can be of little benefit to health.

The new Heart Theory shows that cardiofitness does not develop from calorie amounts of physical activity, as has commonly been assumed. It develops from the same process that improves other muscles, as for example how those in our arms develop from weightlifting. This new theory explains the many previously puzzling research findings about how exercise benefits us.

The really good news is that we do not have to exercise at those high levels to become cardiofit. This book outlines moderate level exercise programs that most people can develop comfortably, which can add seven years of healthy days to life. More important, this can make nearly all those added years better. It is not how long we exercise that counts. I show from overwhelming research that we can get the same or even more benefit from properly walking just 18 minutes each day than from typical walking for an hour or even two hours each day.

Incredibly, we have had no useful way for knowing our all-important cardiofitness level from exercise, or what it accomplishes for us. The new Cardiofitness Ratio, or CFR, described in this book solves this. The CFR correlates results of our exercise directly and with high significance to the risk of most major diseases. I show how you can measure your own CFR from simple treadmill tests. Many should be able to take these tests themselves. Our CFR depends in part on our genetics and in part on our exercise. A poor genetic factor of cardiofitness, which now can be identified, might be a previously unknown time bomb.

I suggest a simple but scientifically-designed new exercise program for nearly everyone called CARDIO 120. This program, requiring just one and a half to two hours a week of exercise, should develop for sedentary people an improvement in cardiofitness from nearly any kind or combination of moderate exercises. Continued faithfully over an extensive time, CARDIO 120 can develop a high level of cardiofitness from an exciting new concept called cardio feed back. CARDIO 120 did this for me.

A sophisticated method called Managed Cardio can help people manage their cardiofitness development from exercise, and show them how to develop nearly any level of desired and achievable cardiofitness. I also introduce a new and simple Cardiofitness Point system that shows how many Points you need to exercise to reach health goals.

This is not a book about bodybuilding or athletics. It gives a new message about how correct exercise can improve our health. It shows how we can waste enormous amounts of time doing exercise that will be of little benefit. It explains and extensively verifies how cardiofitness from moderate exercise can contribute more to our health and longevity than any other now known thing. I hope you will enjoy reading this book, and that it will help you enjoy a longer and better life.

CONTENTS

PART 5

INTRODUCTION

During the early 1970's my company, Exxon (now Exxon Mobil), announced the availability of an exercise program for its executives. Research was showing that proper exercise could reduce the risk of heart attacks. My father had died at age 45 and both grandfathers were gone by 62, all from cardiovascular diseases. I immediately signed up for the program.

We first took a test on a treadmill. It was exhausting. I was so tired out that I could not concentrate the rest of the afternoon. Six months later we took another treadmill test. This one was easy. Puzzled, I asked my doctor what was the purpose of the easy test. He replied, "Forrest, this is the same test you took before!"

I could not believe it! It seemed incredible that a test that had been so exhausting had become so easy after a few months of not difficult regular exercise. I was walking the mile from the commuter train to Rockefeller Center each day faster, and was moving up stairs much faster and easier. I was feeling better and more alive. I now know that this experience was a turning point in my life. I became fascinated with the potential value of regular exercise and have spent much of a following three decades reading, studying, doing research and writing about its importance.

I am a post-graduate chemical engineer and scientific analyst. For most of two decades I headed a group of engineers and scientists that were engaged in full-time analysis of key parts of Exxon's overall research data produced by groups located throughout the world. This highly competent group had pioneered some of the earliest successful use of computers and mathematical methods of analysis that required computers.

I was involved in analyzing complex research not only on chemicals and petroleum but in areas as different as business economics, meteorology, marketing, advertising and health. I was assigned to analyze the research results on what probably was the largest-then research project on the environmental chemical carcinogens that produce cancer. With this background in health research and scientific analysis, I wanted to learn about the exercise I needed to do reduce risk of the disease that had felled my father at such an early age.

The Company Exercise Program

This early program tracked how cardiofitness improved as different kinds and amounts of heart-rate-monitored exercise were done. I use the single word cardiofitness to simplify the tongue-twisting cardiorespiratory fitness now used by researchers. Also, most of what follows in this book is not about respiratory fitness. Cardiofitness directly measures the physical condition of our heart and its associated cardiovascular system. It measures how effectively our heart can distribute blood, oxygen and other nutrients throughout the thousands of miles of arteries, veins and capillaries in this incredible system. The fitness of our cardiovascular system can be far more important to our future health and life than the fitness of any other body muscle.

With help of the project manager I computerized the program data and developed how different exercise heart rates over time produce different levels of cardiofitness. This early program on 265 men for two years may have produced one of the better sets of research data relating exercise heart rates to cardiofitness.

It was obvious even then that higher heart rates during exercise were far more effective in producing cardiofitness than were low heart rates. Cardiofitness did not develop simply from physical activity that is measured by overall calories of exercise. Rather, calories at higher exercise intensity were much more effective than were calories at low level exercise.

After 30 years of more research, scientists are still arguing about the effects of exercise time and intensity on cardiofitness. I see statements like "You don't have to exercise in the gym. Just walk and you will get the same benefit" and "You do not need to do heart-rate exercise; you can get to the same fitness by just living a good lifestyle." This and much other advice about exercise that we hear today is incredible nonsense.

The Early Research

The key question back in the 1970's was: "What benefit does exercise contribute to our health?" The health establishment then was focused on cholesterol and dismissed the role of exercise in reducing risk of heart disease as either nothing or trivial. Having had experience with fallible health research, I visited the medical libraries to learn for myself what the research really had found out about exercise. This project started only as a personal one; I wanted to learn what exercise I needed to do.

I was astounded by the amount of research. Every kind of exercise seemed to reduce heart disease, sometimes very substantially. The few studies that found no effect were of little significance. I ended up with a pile of nearly 50 research papers that included 90 comparisons about exercise and heart disease that nearly all said the same thing: Exercise helps, and more exercise helps more. Keep in mind that this project was done back in the middle 1970's Even then, a lot of research had been done on exercise and health.

I originally assumed that this project would take a couple of weeks. It actually took two full years to read, understand, digest, and seriously analyze the research results in those 50 papers. This may explain why no one else seemed to have seriously analyzed this research.

I was deeply disturbed. How could our health establishment, which is presumed to serve the public interest, claim no or little benefit from exercise in the face of such extensive research findings? This was wrong. Did the establishment confuse something for decades that could have saved or prolonged millions of human lives?

I decided that someone should at least try to tell the truth about the importance of exercise to health, and wrote a book about it. The book was published as The Pulse Point Plan in 1982 with the excellent help of Random House. It was peer-reviewed and introduced by the highly regarded authority on exercise, Dr. Samuel Fox of Georgetown University. The book showed that as above:

The primary health benefit of exercise in reducing risk of heart disease was obtained by improving the physical condition of the heart and cardiovascular system by what we now call cardiofitness. This cardiofitness can be a very important protector of health and life. The physiologists and exercise researchers had been promoting this theory, but it was then uncorroborated. Cardiofitness is measured by an exercise test called "VO2 Max." Values of this measure are of little use to the public because they vary too much for those of different ages and gender.

I proposed a simple index of VO2 Max I now refer to as the Cardiofitness Ratio, or CFR. The CFR approximates the ratio of a person's VO2 Max to an average population VO2 Max for age and gender. The ratio is multiplied by 100 to develop whole numbers rather than decimal numbers. A CFR of 100 refers to an average cardiofitness for age and gender. A CFR of say 120 directly shows a cardiofitness that is much better than and 20% higher than usual for age. A CFR of 80 immediately reveals a very deficient cardiofitness that shows a high health risk.

During the 1970's physiologists and other researchers were promoting the cardiofitness theory and advising rather vigorous heart-rate-monitored exercise. An opposing group claimed that benefits of exercise were related simply to calories of exercise done. No study had been published as of that decade that directly measured the effect of cardiofitness on the risk of heart disease or any other disease.

I thus examined every published study in depth, and estimated the likely differences in both exercise calories and cardiofitness in CFR of the groups that exercised and those that did not exercise. This was a tiresome task that took months to complete. The results were overwhelmingly significant.

There was no useful relation between calories of exercise and risk of heart disease. In contrast, cardiofitness seemed to explain remarkably well the results obtained from the fifty useful data sets from the research on exercise and heart disease published before 1980. Differences in risk of heart disease ranging up to more than five times were clearly explained by differences in cardiofitness. This study published in my 1982 book provided (as noted in the Prologue) what I feel was a first scientific confirmation that cardiofitness is the key exercise factor that protects against heart disease.

The first studies of risk as related to actually measured amounts of cardiofitness started to become available in 1983, about 5 years after my work for the book had been done. These studies confirmed almost exactly my work that had established a relationship of cardiofitness reducing the risk of heart disease. I reproduce results of my first analysis and results of those early and subsequent studies in Appendix 7.

This was enormously exciting! It confirmed that the relationship between exercise defined by the CFR of cardiofitness and heart disease was scientifically fundamental and casual. Health research nearly always compares results on two or more groups of people that do different things. Such studies usually show only associations that may or may not have useful value. A Holy Grail of research is to forecast a relationship from scientific theory that is later found to be correct by direct measurement. The Cardiofitness Ratio, or CFR, met this difficult test.

Starting about 1995 a major change was made in recommendations for exercise. The former concept of cardiofitness and heart-rate-monitored exercise was suddenly abandoned and people were advised mostly to walk 30 minutes daily. A recent update of the advice made in 2007 did suggest doing some "vigorous" exercise, but again there was no adequate recognition of cardiofitness. More about this later.

Today's Confusion

Sadly, I feel that the entire subject of exercise and health is now in disarray. The idea that exercise is important is no longer controversial. A mass of research shows exercise to be increasingly important. But the public still has not been provided a really useful guide as to what amount and kind of exercise will produce little, good, or excellent health benefits. Every article on health today admonishes you to exercise. This really tells us nothing very useful.

Most books about exercise have been entitled Physical Activity. This is the wrong focus. Amounts of physical activity can have little to do with the exercise that produces cardiofitness. Thousands of calories per day of occupational physical activity can produce only very small improvements in cardiofitness. Just 125 calories or only 30 minutes a week of the correct exercise can produce a better cardio benefit.

People today, including doctors and health professionals, still do not know their level of cardiofitness by a measure such as the CFR. Our health establishment has evidenced little interest in helping our population measure their cardiofitness or understand what it can mean to them.

Global Analysis of Exercise Done for this Book is Different

Today's research on the benefits of our health habits is a world of statistics and statistical associations. Each study produces a statistical ratio of a disease suffered by two groups that do something differently. These study statistics have high error margins. Health experts usually try to develop conclusions and yo-yo their advice by looking mostly at just some of the more recent of these studies. Such statistics suggest things that may be good to do, but they fail to tell us what we need to do to get a useful benefit.

Global Scientific Analysis uses the methods of engineering and physical science to probe more deeply into the entire body of available research. Global Analysis aims to learn more about and quantify the underlying mechanisms. These more sophisticated analyses show far more accurately how we really need to exercise to obtain useful reductions in the risk of major diseases. They also show that much advice on how to exercise has been seriously wrong.

Chapters 2 and 3 provide specific examples of Global Scientific Analysis that organize results from available research on how cardiofitness reduces risk of heart disease. These analyses convert often confusing statistics to values that can be understood and used by people. Global Scientific

Analysis often provides a new and exciting view of what research has really learned. Important and fascinating new findings are specifically revealed in these and following chapters, were not found by the original researchers.

Each new finding about exercise and cardiofitness in this book is verified either in peer-reviewed papers or in my papers published at http://www.lifeahead.net. Each major finding in this book is demonstrated and confirmed by an analysis of most or all of the actual available research results. Many of these papers include the actual research data.

Proper and adequate exercise can substantially reduce our risk of heart attack, cancer, and other major diseases. But no exercise or diet or other health habit can completely prevent a disease. But I suggest to use the advice of your doctor in planning your exercise. If good exercise habits do not prevent a major disease from happening, they probably will defer this event for many years.

Part One in the book shows how the kinds and amounts of exercise develop measured levels of cardiofitness and protection of our health. As example, I show how different levels of walking pace and duration done each week reduce our health risk. Incredibly, and despite all of the talk about walking for health, I find no evidence that this seemingly elementary analysis has ever been properly done and published. These results should shock many in the world of exercise. I show for the first time in the Master Tables how exercising at different levels will produce specific levels of cardiofitness and improvements in health. These results also will surprise the experts.

The new CARDIO 120 program shows how you can develop desirable goals and possibly even very high goals for cardiofitness from a variety of moderate exercise programs. Managed Cardio shows you the exercise times and heart rates needed to reach any feasible cardiofitness goal. The new and simple Cardiofitness Point method shows how you can exercise usefully and move toward really useful goals for health.

Part Two shows how cardiofitness can reduce risk of major diseases and death far more than has been previously realized. It shows from extensive but easy to understand scientific analysis how our level of cardiofitness may be more important to our future health and life than is any other major health risk factor.

Part Three tells much more about the fascinating measure of our cardiofitness called the CFR. As example, how it can differ for populations and how it has changed historically, with age, with lifestyle, and with exercise. Few people have known their cardiofitness because existing tests have been too demanding and expensive. I describe new simple tests for measuring your CFR that nearly everyone should be able to take. Everyone should know his or her CFR and what it means.

Part Four tells the truth about some exercise associations that have been a source of recent controversy. These include the effect of different kinds of exercise on body weight; and the health benefit of resistance-type exercise and the health value for doing the new fad of Step Counts.

Part Five answers many questions people have had about their exercise. It shows some of the many additional benefits of exercise found in research. I tell more about the many exercises that can produce your cardiofitness and their advantages and shortcomings. I suggest some facts and ideas that I hope can help motivate you to do your exercise regularly.

Appendix sections provide the guides that show you how to exercise effectively, how to take the new tests for cardiofitness, and how the free Life Ahead computer program on the internet can help you establish exercise goals and benefits. It tells more about how exercise develops its health benefits, and provides further scientific support of some key new ideas in the book. Chapter 1 tells about the research we now have on exercise that shows the remarkable importance to our health and life of our cardiofitness.

Part One

Cardiofitness Is The Key.

How To Achieve Any Desired Goal For Cardiofitness

CHAPTER 1

The Research on Exercise, Cardiofitness and Health

Some History

For hundreds of generations men and women have been physically active throughout their entire lives. 40% of the US population lived and worked on small farm as late as at the turn of the 20th century. Farm machinery was the horse, and those on farms worked from dawn to dusk Most of our population worked in occupations that required physical labor. People walked to work, to shops, and to the homes of others during the days before the automobile. At the start of the 20th century coronary heart disease – today the #1 killer of our population – was unknown to most doctors. In those earlier days most people generated enough exercise from their daily living to protect themselves from the high risks that people have today. And few people then smoked cigarettes.

Heart disease grew rapidly during the early years of the 20th century. By the 1930's disturbing numbers of men were suddenly dropping dead. This could happen when they were exerting themselves as in shoveling snow or digging in the garden. It thus seemed obvious to doctors that exercise increased risk of heart disease. Those who recovered from an attack were advised to get plenty of bed rest and to avoid exercise. This medical advice that is now known to be false continued during and well beyond the first half of the century.

That First and Now Classic Study

Epidemiologist Dr. Jerry Morris noticed in the late 1940's that the drivers of the London buses seemed to be having many more attacks than did the conductors that stood and walked about all day. Concerned, he organized the statistics and found in 1949 that the drivers were getting twice as many attacks as the conductors. Morris knew that this would not then be taken as credible because so many doctors had assumed that exercise was bad for the heart. He thus developed other evidence and waited until November of 1953 to publish with co-workers a landmark research study of the 20th century, "Coronary Heart Disease and the Physical Activity of Work."[2]

The paper included three separate studies. First, of the 90 deaths from heart disease from 17,000 bus men, the drivers suffered twice as frequently as did the conductors who walked about most of the day. Second, of 314 heart attack deaths from 62,000 postal employees, the less active workers suffered 1.9 times as many heart attacks as did the mail carriers that walked most of the day. And third, of 3.5 million male workers throughout England and Wales in an earlier year the coronary disease deaths rates per 100,000 were 856 for light physical workers, 550 for those having intermediate activity, and 396 for the heavy physical workers.

The results on the bus men were barely significant. But the results on the much larger group of postal workers was significant at above 500 to 1. And the results from all workers in the country were very significant.

Dr. Morris's study was ignored in Britain and outraged many in the US medical establishment. The idea that physical activity that experts knew to be risky could actually be healthy seemed preposterous. Negative claims were widespread such as the larger trouser size of the drivers might have been involved. (This was absurd.) Or that the stress of driving caused the drivers' attacks

Discussion always was about the bus drivers and conductors, who were the smallest of the three included population groups, and few critics seemed to have ever read the paper. For example, the postmen and other workers had no associated stress of driving. Morris said later that he should have published the three studies in three successive papers rather than to wait and include them in just one paper. But a number of US researchers – mostly the physiologists – were fascinated.

Another study of the bus conductors and drivers in 1966 by Morris[3] showed the same results for many more drivers and conductors studied between 1956 and 1960, and for train conductors and motormen. In 1973 he published landmark research on the benefits of leisure time exercise.[4] In 1990 he published another important study of leisure time exercise and coronary disease on 9300 British civil workers over 9 years.[5] He found excellent benefits for fast walking, but little benefit for average pace walking. He showed that unless exercise was at least fairly vigorous it provided small if any reduction in heart disease. He also noted that calories of exercise did not explain risk of heart disease.

People Became Involved

Few people in the US exercised for health before about 1970. The idea that exercise was good was accepted. But few realized what the automobile and a vast introduction of mechanical aids had done to their physical condition. In 1968 Kenneth Cooper's now classic book Aerobics became a top seller. Many mostly middle-age and younger men started to get their "30 Aerobic Points" of exercise that Cooper showed would make them cardiofit. It became increasingly popular to go to the gym.

Aerobic dancing became popular and thousands of these programs were being enjoyed by women across the US starting in the 1970's. Jogging and running also became popular. Most people who continued good aerobic exercise could feel the way their physical condition had improved. Fortunately, despite the apparent lack of support for this excellent exercise by many of today's so-called health experts, much of it continues to this day.

The Physical Activity of Work

In spite of nearly 50 exercise research studies published before 1980, most of our medical establishment remained immune to the results of research on exercise and physical activity. The tiresome repetitive reply was "It isn't proved." Most heart researchers then were working on cholesterol. In 1976 I wrote in cooperation with a professor from the University of Pennsylvania a substantial paper for publication in a scientific journal. This paper cited the important research results then published on heart disease and exercise, and showed that the key casual factor that protected us from the disease appeared to be cardiovascular fitness. The paper was returned by a reviewer with a scrawl saying "How about Cholesterol? Do not Publish." The BIG

THING then was diet and cholesterol, and many researchers that controlled peer review view a paper on another subject as an intrusion into their message. The reviewer obviously did not even read the paper because it actually did include a section about how exercise improved cholesterol.

Most early research on physical activity was for men in different occupations. This included results for farmers vs. urban dwellers, and others on longshoremen, railroad section men, postal carriers, and utility workers. An average usual benefit from these occupation studies was about a reduction in risk of 1.5 to 2 times. But it seemed likely that the more active workers consumed a typical 3,000-6,000 more calories of physical activity per work week than did the inactive workers. A criticism of this early research was that it produced little guidance for people. A person hardly would change occupation to become a mail carrier or longshoreman just to reduce risk of a disease. The key implication of Morris's research was that perhaps leisure time physical activity also could be beneficial.

The Research on Leisure Time Exercise

The physiologists were not disturbed by this large requirement of physical activity calories for health benefit. The predominant early theory was that exercise benefits the heart, and much physiological research on what we now call cardiofitness had been done. It was known that the physical capability of the heart was improved most effectively by vigorous exercise at significantly elevated heart rates. Exercise at heart rates much below 100 per minute produced little benefit to cardiofitness. Industrial workers that suffered heart attacks rarely obtained much higher heart rates than this.

A first really useful study of leisure time activity by Sam Shapiro of the New York Health Insurance Plan was published in 1969. Although omitted in most reviews of exercise research, I found this 60 page study fascinating. It showed that risks of heart disease for those that did not exercise were about 2 times higher for those that were physically active either on the job, or in their leisure time. Those most active both on the job and in leisure had a risk of heart disease reduced by 3.3 times. But risks for a sudden death from coronary disease ranged up to 20 times for low amounts of leisure time activity, and risk of a sudden death for physically inactive smokers could be even higher.

A BIG THING here was that leisure time physical activity produced a substantial reduction in the risk of heart disease that was at least equal to that from heavy occupational physical activity that probably involved far more energy calories. Shapiro's very large study which included more than 400 disease or death events on 32,000 people, was of extremely high significance. Morris's 1973 study showed that leisure time exercise could produce a substantial difference in risks. Those having some exercise at a good intensity level of 7.5 kcal per minute obtained about one-third of the heart disease of those that did little exercise.

Ralph Paffenbarger published a study of Harvard University alumni in 1978. This showed that the graduates doing the least exercise had a risk of 1.7 times for heart attack and 2 times for heart attack death. This became an instant best seller in the US for the proponents of exercise. For some reason many that had overlooked the prior studies of Morris and Shapiro found this to be something really new.

Paffenbarger cited a demanding 2,000 calories per week as a target for exercise, and suggested an exercise intensity goal of 7.5 calories per minute. If most of this activity was done at a suggested intensity level of 7.5 calories per minute, this would produce excellent benefits. But rather few would adopt such a program and as before, calories is not a useful basis for planning exercise. Ralph Paffenbarger made major contributions in supporting the importance of exercise to health. He was a proponent of and later published papers on the benefits of cardiofitness.

The Landmark Study of Cardiovascular Fitness

The final study I will discuss – the most important of exercise in the 20th century – was that of the Cooper Institute in Dallas. In November of 1989 Steven Blair with others published the paper "Physical Fitness and All-Cause Mortality." This study showed extraordinary risks of cardiovascular diseases, cancer and death from all causes to be associated with different amounts of cardiofitness. Figure 1-1 shows the major health risks of poor cardiofitness in ratio to those of high fitness found in this landmark study.

The highest bars in Figure 1-1 shows that the risks of cardiovascular diseases were 8 to 9 times higher for both men (M) and women (W) of low cardiofitness than for those of high cardiofitness. Those of moderate cardiofitness developed about a three times higher risk than those of high cardiofitness. As before, the measure of cardiofitness I use in this book is called cardiofitness ratio, or CFR. An average CFR of men and women is 100, and the unfit groups of men and women in this research had about a 90 CFR, or a cardiofitness 90% of that of average. The moderate fitness group had a CFR of about 110, and the high cardiofitness groups had a

Figure 1-1

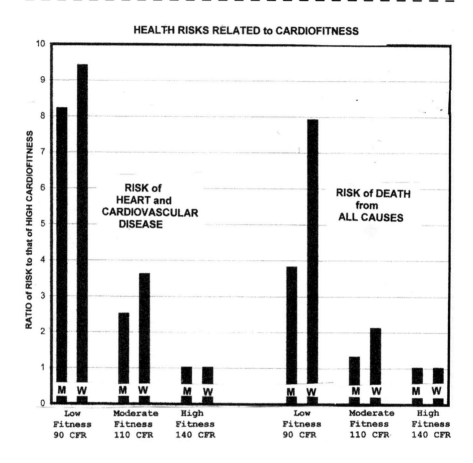

HEALTH RISKS RELATED to CARDIOFITNESS

quite high cardiofitness of about 140 CFR or 140% of average for age and gender. The bars at the right show that risk of death from all diseases and other causes was an extraordinary 4 to 8 times higher for unfit men and women than for those that were quite fit.

The authors showed that these differences were related to another direct measure of cardiofitness called "metabolic equivalents." The high fitness groups had a capability of 10 or more metabolic equivalents that was more than 50% higher than the 6 metabolic equivalents of the low fitness groups. The researchers kindly provided me the information needed to compute the values of the CFR.

The striking finding from this and study of cardiofitness was the enormous differences of risk involved. Most studies of exercise found differences in risk of 1.5 to 2 times, not 4 to 8 times. Differences in risk of heart disease associated with different diet factors typically develop differences of 1.5 times or less. People today think about exercise as some generality that is good. This difference in risk for cardiofitness identifies something extraordinarily different than just good. This study also showed that very high reductions in risk of cancer also were developed from increased cardiofitness. The high fitness men had a 4.3 times lower risk of cancer and the high fitness women had more than a ten times lower risk of all types of cancer.

Low Cardiofitness Identifies a Serious Health Risk:

Most publicity about cardiofitness has been about how higher values from exercise reduce heart risk. Yet the most important finding of Blair's study may have been the extremely high risks associated with low values of cardiofitness. I will show later that risks of heart disease associated with low cardiofitness can be twice or three times as high as average, and ten times higher than those with good cardiofitness. Most men and women today that do no regular exercise have a CFR of about 90, or close to that of the above men and women that had the highest risk of heart disease and premature death in the Cooper Institute study.

Now please note carefully from the above chart how the moderate fitness groups obtained most of the reduction in risk of heart disease and death from all causes. The high fitness groups of a 140 CFR included the many that were out running many miles everyday. But just a moderate cardiofitness of 110 CFR developed the largest reduction in risk, and especially that for risk of death from all causes. I will show throughout this book that you do not have to exercise at those very high levels to obtain most of the health benefit of exercise. You really have to move your cardiofitness up 20% from a below average value of 90 to an above average value of 110 to get the largest benefit to your health. I call this improvement of 20% in cardiofitness a "Good" objective for your exercise. Much of this book focuses on how you can develop that objective with a minimum of time and effort.

You do not have to do that very high intensity level of exercise to reach the Good target for your CFR. But you will not get there by just some ordinary walking 30 minutes every day or from some gardening and golf. You do need to develop a scientifically-designed program of moderate exercise and usually need to do this moderate exercise for about two hours each week.

Calories of Exercise Again Do Not Explain Cardiofitness

The physical activity calories usual in this Blair study were quoted as 200 per week for the inactive group of men and 1650 for the more active and cardiofit groups of men. For reference, Paffenbarger obtained a 1.7 times risk of heart disease for men from 2000 calories per week of ordinary exercise. Blair's study found a 7.9 times risk in heart disease for measured cardiofitness from a difference of only 1450 calories per week of exercise. Cardiofitness thus produced at least a five times larger reduction in risk from a smaller difference in calories of exercise than was obtained by Paffenbarger's physical activity calories. This is one of many examples illustrating the far greater importance of cardiofitness to risk than is associated with physical activity calories of exercise.

This and other evidence suggest that 100 exercise calories of efficient cardio exercise will develop the overall health benefits of about 600 calories of what usually is identified as ordinary physical activity. A similar factor from other measurements, which I will discuss later, suggests that about 85% of all health benefits from physical activity and exercise will be developed by cardio-effective exercise. This again suggests about a six-fold difference in health-effectiveness of cardio vs. other physical activity calories.

Despite this and much other impressive direct evidence about the health effectiveness of exercise, much of our exercise research community still seems to be lost in the wilderness of physical activity. We see exercise recommendations based on physical activity, seminars on physical activity, and books about physical activity. This provides a focus on what at maximum is only one-sixth of what is really important about exercise.

From a physical science view, these vast differences in health risk of 5 to 10 times vs.1.5 to 2 times for similar amounts of physical activity calories are extremely exciting. The question becomes, "What mechanism can explain these fascinating results?" This is a question of enormous importance to the health of our public. Without cardiofitness, we have no mechanism that can explain a difference in risk of death of up to many times for both men and women.

I have pondered this question for much of twenty-five years. I believe that it is now mostly answered. The new Heart Theory I will outline later does provide a simple and straightforward answer to this fascinating and important problem of how cardiofitness develops from exercise. It explains results of much research that previously was contradictory and confusing. It has vitally important implications about how we need to exercise to improve our health.

The Cooper Institute group headed by Steven Blair has published dozens of other studies which show in different ways the importance of cardiofitness. Of particular importance was their study showing how the heart disease of groups that stopped exercising increased, and how that of others that started to exercise diminished within just a very few years.

Others Have Shown the Importance of Cardiovascular Fitness

The Cooper Institute study was not the only study and was not even the first that showed this dramatic importance of cardiofitness. This finding is confirmed by at least nine other studies.

A striking verification of cardiofitness and risk of heart disease also came from a study by Gustavo Arraiz and co-workers.[7] They measured the physical activity of each of a representative population sample of 8,800 Canadians. Each in the study answered a detailed questionnaire about his or her physical activity, and was tested by a fairly simple home fitness test. No relationship with cardiovascular diseases was found between the very active, active, moderate and physically inactive groups identified by questionnaires about their physical activity. Yet incredibly, the 992 people that did not pass the fitness test had a risk of cardiovascular disease 5.3 times higher than did a similar size group that passed the minimum acceptable level of this test!

Arraiz thus showed that specific types of physical activity produced cardiofitness and health benefits. These types of physical activity were not recognized by conventional questions about calorie amounts of exercise. Much of what has traditionally thought to be physical activity and that is measured by calories produces little cardiofitness benefit.

Other research studies that found similar large effects of cardiofitness on risks of heart disease and premature death were by Ekelund,[8] Sobolski,[9] and Lie.[10] Physical activity related only minimally to risk. But differences in measured cardiofitness always seemed to reveal very high relationships with risk. This and many other studies found that more physical activity calories did not produce much gain in health. It required increased cardiofitness.

Table 1-1 shows the risk ratios of cardiovascular disease from the 10 available studies relating risk to actually measured values of cardiofitness.[79] The unfit persons obtained from 2.3 to 9.9 times the risk of those more cardiofit. The two left columns in this table identify and reference the studies found and show their size, gender and location. The right column shows the risk of cardiovascular disease for poor cardiofitness group divided by the risk of cardiovascular disease for the good cardiofitness group. The third column shows the differences in cardiofitness of the groups studied as measured by the CFR

The BIG THING in Table 1-1 is the very large difference in ratios of risk of disease for those groups having the higher levels of difference in CFR. The average risk ratio for the six studies that measured the benefit of CFR differences of 24 or higher was 7.7. This means that the risk of disease for the poor cardiofitness group was 7.7 times higher than was the risk of the good cardiofitness group. This value of above 7 again dwarfs the usual risk of about 1.5 to 2 times obtained in dozens of studies of physical

Table 1-1

Table 1-1 Studies of Cardiovascular Disease Risk vs Differences in Measured Cardiofitness in CFR			
Study Author And Date	Study Size And Country	Est Diff in CFR	Risk Ratio, Low fitness to high fitness
Peters[11], 1983	2800 Men	18	2.5
Lie[10],1985	2800 Men, Norway	33	6.7
Sobolski[9], 1987	2900 Men, Belgium	30	7.7
Ekelund[8], 1988	3100 Men, US & Canada	24	8.3
Blair[6], 1989	10200 Men US	29	7.7
	3100 Women	37	9.9
Arraiz[7] 1992	8700 Men in Canada	22	5.3
Hein[12], 1992	5000 Men, Denmark	40	5.9
Sandvick[13] 1993	1960 Men, Norway	19	3.3
Lakka[14] 1994	1166 Men in Finland	19	2.3
Mora[15] 2003	3000 Women US	22	2.9

activity such as the one of Paffenbarger mentioned above. As before, the CFR simply approximates the ratio of measured cardiofitness by VO2 Max to that average for age and gender. In fact, if we relate risks of disease and death first to differences measured in cardiofitness, we can find no further effect of calories of physical activity.

I have provided in Appendix 7 results of much more research that demonstrates further the important effect of cardiofitness for those interested. It now seems likely that the health value of all or at least nearly all of what researchers have called 'physical activity' or 'exercise' really is due to amounts of cardiofitness.

Can we as individuals develop the cardiofitness needed to reduce risk of heart disease by 7 or more times? Studies that I will describe later have shown that many groups of men and women have achieved improvements in CFR and VO2 of 20-25% or more from fairly vigorous exercise in about 6 months. These improvements probably can also be obtained from moderate exercise performed over a longer term. The average reduction in risk of heart disease for a CFR differences of 20% is about 3.5 times. Each improvement of 1% in cardiofitness maintained over life will reduce risk of heart disease by 6.4% and add about one-third of a year to our expectancy of healthy days of life. An added 20 or 20% to our CFR could thus give us about 7 more estimated years of healthy life.

The above men and women that obtained 20-25% improvements in CFR probably would obtain gains of 25-30 CFR gains after a year of exercise. And those that develop serious cardio-exercise can obtain gains in cardiofitness of above 40%. More about this is discussed later.

A logical question from every health-interested person becomes, "How do I have to exercise to obtain this very attractive gain of this 6-7 more years of healthy days of life?" Can I obtain it from walking? Or do I have to run or use the treadmill? Answers to questions like this that have not previously been available will be provided in the chapters that follow.

The Cooper Institute showed that nearly 50% of the men in their high cardiofitness and lowest risk of disease group had been jogging or running, 20% had been exercising on the treadmill, and 12% had been using the exercise bicycle. About 21% of women had been jogging or running, and 23% had been doing aerobic dancing. These are the usual kinds of exercise that over time can produce the high CFR of 140 measured for these groups. In contrast, most in the low fitness and high risk groups were doing minimal or no exercise.

Incredibly, these striking differences have been and still are being largely ignored by our present health establishment. For the health statistician these values are just more numbers to be averaged together with all other risk ratio numbers for 'exercise.' To the physical scientist they are a striking and exciting finding and a monumental discovery that requires a seriously developed explanation. Health-interested people that want to protect their health and life will logically ask, "What do I have to do to obtain these large benefits?"

Risk differences for a major health factor ranging up to 6 to 9 times are extraordinary. It requires a 400 total serum cholesterol to reach a 6.5 times risk vs. an average person's cholesterol of about 215. Only a tiny few people have a 400 or higher total cholesterol. But a far larger number of today's middle-age and younger men and women can have a 5 or 6 times higher than average risk of heart disease by having a very low cardiofitness.

Chapter 7 following shows more about the strikingly important risks of heart disease, cancer, diabetes, dementia and other major diseases that are associated with cardiofitness. Appendix 7 tells more about the monumental evidence supporting the importance of cardiofitness.

I mentioned in the introduction that exercise recommendations starting in the early 1970's and prior to about 1995 were based on the concept of cardiofitness and did recommend heart-rate-targeted exercise that might effectively reduce risks of heart and other important diseases. These recommendations typically advised 15-30 minutes on each of 3 to 5 days per week of moderate to high heart-rate-monitored exercise. But during much of this time, many in the health establishment still were contesting a health benefit of exercise.

The Surgeon General Issues a Report

During 1996 – after 40 years of argument– the benefits of exercise on health were finally endorsed by the US Surgeon General.[17] The report included a mass of valuable information including the statistical risk ratios found in more than a hundred studies. It showed that exercise protected against a wide variety of diseases. But the title of the report and much of its content talked about 'physical activity' as the assumed primary cause.

The report recommends that people of all ages should do a minimum 30 minutes of moderate exercise such as brisk walking on all or most days of the week and says, "More exercise can be better." But I find no mention about what benefit this amount of walking might produce. And their recommendation about what exercise the public should do represented a major shift from the official recommendations that had prevailed during the previous decades. There was no recommendation to do what we now call cardio or fairly vigorous exercise. Recommendations of other official committees repeated this recommendation but with more emphasis on walking as the moderate exercise.

Incredibly, nine of the ten studies in Table 1-1 that showed the remarkable benefits of cardiofitness had been published when the Surgeon General's report was released. I find no mention of the extraordinary benefits found by these studies. I also fail to find any useful published research that verifies the health value of walking 30 minutes each day at the time these new recommendations were made.

How Could this Shift in Exercise Recommendations Happen?

Many experts were concerned that exercise at high heart rates was not appropriate or acceptable to many in our older population who most needed exercise. More vigorous exercise such as running increases injuries. These concerns led many to oppose the recommendations that everyone should do

14

what was presumed to be high heart rate exercise. There also was the possibility that more people could be encouraged to do lower-level exercise than would do higher-level exercise. This led to strong arguments among anti-fitness and pro-fitness groups about the best type of exercise to propose.

The 1996 Recommendation on Walking Was an Unfortunate Mistake

Considering the evidence available at that time, a recommendation that many people should do 'moderate' exercise was appropriate. But I feel that a first serious error was the omission of a more effective alternative of doing more vigorous exercise. There was no apparent consideration of the key factor of cardiofitness. This effectively left the more useful potential of cardio exercise as unsupported. A second error was the absence of any useful measure of exercise intensity such as an exercise heart rate. And a third error was the lack of any adequate direct research then – and even now – that specifically supports the benefits of walking or other moderate exercise of 3 to 3.5 hours or more every week. This large duration of needed exercise time placed a serious time burden on our population and probably has discouraged many from exercising. I show later that a need for this duration of exercise is not now verified by research.

This 1996 Recommendation implied to many that "Vigorous exercise is not needed." Or even that "Vigorous exercise was not recommended." Or that "30 minutes every day of walking is the excellent and ultimate exercise program." The key word 'brisk' that is too vague to be a useful monitor of exercise intensity was often omitted in translations of this advice. These implications simply were not true.

A reading of many wellness newsletters and articles about exercise reveals that the potential value for doing good cardio exercise has been forgotten by many health experts during the past decade. This was not intended by the Surgeon General report that says, "It is acknowledged that for most people, greater health benefits can be obtained by engaging in physical activity of more vigorous intensity or of longer duration."

Fortunately, those earlier recommendations to exercise at say 50% to 90% of maximum heart rate were not forgotten. They continued to display on the website of the American College of Sports Medicine. Millions of people are still doing what is called good cardio by using in part these prior recommendations as reference. Many of these people still doing productive cardio exercise never have heard about this lack of official support for this exercise. But as I will discuss later, the recommendations about doing exercise at certain percentages of maximum heart rate are seriously flawed and need a substantial update. We do not have to do the high-intensity exercise that was implied as needed in some pre-1996 advice.

A New Update Recommendation Is Better

In November of 2007 an update recommendation about exercise was published by a Committee of the American College of Sports Medicine and the American Heart Association.[83,84] Appearing with a near fanfare, two exercise update papers for differing age groups were published nearly simultaneously by two respected medical journals. The new papers proposed two levels of exercise called Moderate-Intensity Aerobic and Vigorous-Intensity. As a minimum, a person of any age could do either Moderate-Intensity exercise for 2½ hours per week or Vigorous-Intensity exercise for one hour each week, or mixtures of these exercises.

This new proposal corrects what was the most serious error in the 1996 recommendation by acknowledging the benefits of vigorous exercise. Also, the times required are more accurate representations of results of actual research than are the excessive times asked for in earlier proposals. These new general guides identify what from today's research could be a minimum but not necessarily a desirable exercise for most health-interested adults. The words 'brisk' and 'vigorous' supplemented by a confusing 200-word description for exercise intensity can be interpreted quite differently by individual people.

No estimate of a benefit was shown in this proposal. I estimate that people attempting to follow this advice would develop widely varying benefits with an average improvement of perhaps 7% in cardiofitness. This would reduce risk of heart disease by an average of about 1.5 times. But many, from their interpretations of what was moderate and vigorous, would develop much lesser benefit. This compares with goals I will propose of 10% from cardiofitness and 1.85 times reduction in heart disease for first goal and 20% and 3.5 times for a good goal from more accurately developed and monitored moderate exercise.

As mentioned in the Prologue, you deserve a more accurately defined and more broadly based minimum program for exercising for health. You also deserve advice for developing much more healthful exercise programs than just a minimum program.

Cardiofitness Is in Disarray and Being Forgotten

I continue to be concerned about the lack of scientific focus in these recommendations. It is not just exercise, it is not just physical activity, and it is not just calories that mostly benefit health. It is cardiofitness. Cardiofitness is a direct measurement of the health and capability of the most important organs in our body – our heart and its accompanying cardiovascular system.

Cardiofitness is a health factor everyone should know about. It is a health factor every doctor should know about a patient. The chapters that follow tell what you can do to develop and maintain a healthful cardiofitness. The all important first subject is, "How much can walking improve our future health?"

CHAPTER 2

Walking and Heart Disease

If you have not been exercising regularly you usually should start by walking more. As we become older walking may be our main exercise. Proper walking can produce aerobic exercise and good health benefits. Sadly, much walking done today for health probably is producing inadequate health benefits. We have excellent direct research on the health benefits of walking that tells us what we need to do. But incredibly, no one seems to have studied this research comprehensively and provided their results to the public!

We've been told again and again that we should walk a half hour (The Institute of Medicine says a full hour) every day for our health. A person today may have 16 hours day awake. But subtract time for dressing, eating, commuting to and from work, time at work, and other time needed for essential tasks and the time left for things we most like to do may be only 2 to 3 hours each day. The demand for a full hour or even a half hour of this time is a considerable request. It is a request that can keep a sizeable part of our population from doing any exercise.

We need to practice good health habits for our entire life. These habits become increasingly important as we get older because our health risks move higher as age moves higher. Logical questions are "What benefit will I achieve from this? If I walk half as much time will I get benefits? If so, how much less? Does spending the considerable time that is recommend for exercise really pay off? Could I get better benefits from some other kind of exercise in lesser time spent?"

I find no useful published answer to any of these questions. It seems to have been assumed that moderate exercise from some research exercise did produce health benefits, and that walking was moderate exercise.

Let Us See What the Research on Walking Really Shows

We now have good research on walking and risk of heart disease. A global analysis of this research that follows answers previously unanswered questions. Ten studies are found published on the risk of heart disease for different walking durations and walking paces.

Table 2-1 shows at right the approximate maximum benefits in reducing risk of heart disease obtained in each of these studies. The columns at left show the author, size and location of the studies.

The typical maximum high/low risk ratio for heart disease found from these studies of walking was about 2 times. This compares with a 5.7 times average benefit from the higher cardiofitness groups shown in Table 1-1. Although this benefit from highest amounts of actual walking researched is smaller than that from best cardiofitness, I will show later that a benefit of 2.0 times still is a very useful health benefit

The average reductions in risk in these research studies were well below the maximum benefit values from walking noted in Table 2-1. We need to know what kind and amount of walking produced the benefits. I thus organized all of the available research on walking to investigate how the pace of walking and duration of walking each week reduced the risk of heart disease.

The results showed a consistent and highly significant relationship between the pace and risk. Each increase in walking pace of one mile per hour up to 4.5 miles per hour reduced risk of heart disease by about 20 percent. This result was as expected and was similar to that concluded by the various researchers

But the Effect of Walking Duration is Very Different!

Incredibly, most of the research showed only small and confusing effects of walking duration on risk of heart disease! The average benefit of walking duration in hours per week in reducing risk of heart disease from a meta analysis of all of the 62 measurements recorded in the above ten studies was small and of dubious significance. How could this be?

Researchers long have assumed that walking pace and walking duration had similar benefits on health and could be inter-changeable. That is, we could walk at a fast pace for a given time or a slower pace at a longer time and obtain the same benefit. I believe that every researcher, health expert, and others involved in health – including me – has assumed that more walking and more exercise each week is better

Yet two of the studies of walking involved research on mail carriers in the US and England that were estimated to walk about 30 hours each week. The carriers obtained a similar reduction in risk of heart disease as did those that walked only two hours each week. Long durations of walking in most studies produced little if any more benefit than did much shorter durations. How could this happen? An answer to this puzzle was finally found:

Table 2-1

Table 2-1 Studies of Walking on the Risk of Cardiovascular Disease		
Study Author Gender, (M) or (F)	Study Size	Max Risk Ratio High / Low
1. Morris[2], 1953, (M)	61,000 postal carriers, Britain	1.9
2. Kahn[21], HA, (M)	Mail Carriers, US 62,000 person years	2.8
3. Morris[5], 1990, (M)	9,400 men in Britain	1.9
4. LaCroix[22], 1996, (M)	1645 in Canada, Age 65+	1.3
Same (F)	Age 65+	2.2
5. Hakim[23], 1998 (M)	700 non-smoking Age 61-81 in Hawaii	3.3
6 Manson[24] 1999 (F)	72,500 Nurses in US age 50+ fastest pace	1.6
7. Lee 2001[25] (F)	39,000 Health Professionals US	1.9
8. Tanasescu[26] 2002 (M)	44,500 US Health Professionals fast pace	2.0
9. Manson[27], 2002 (F)	73,700 Women's Health Initiative US	2.0
10. Noda[28], 2005 (M & F)	31,000 men and 42,000 women in Japan	1.8

Walking for durations up to about 2 hours per week at a given pace and exercise intensity reduces risk of heart disease as expected. Walking similarly for amounts beyond 2 hours per does not reduce this risk further

This discovery is both new and shocking. Nearly every 'expert' recommendation about exercise has told us that we should walk at least 30 minutes nearly every day and from 3 1/2 to 7 hours per week. Yet nearly every useful research study on walking shows no further reduction in risk of heart disease for walking in excess of two hours per week! This was not just ordinary research. It included multiple results from our largest and most respected studies of up to 70,000 persons. Have millions been mostly wasting time doing vast amounts of exercise that produce near zero health benefit?

It is rare that such consistent results for any health factor are found for 9 out of 10 different mostly major studies. To investigate this finding even more intensively I organized all 62 measurements of risk of heart disease included in the above available ten key studies of walking and heart disease in order of duration of walking. The first hour of average walking pace reduced risk 23%. The first two hours of average walking reduced risk 38%. This suggested that the 2nd hour produced a further average reduction of 15% in risk above that developed for the first hour of walking. The third hour produced no further gain. More hours up to 10 per week and the mail carriers 30 hours per week produced no further significant benefit. More evidence about this highly significant finding is in Appendix 3 and in the reference paper on my website.[20]

This confirmed two-hour limit throws another bombshell into present thinking about exercise: Most present and past concepts – including mine – about how exercise improves cardiofitness and reduces risk of heart disease must have been wrong. Physical or chemical processes nearly always proceed continuously and orderly in response to casual factors. It seems logical that more exercise should produce a further benefit. Benefits usually should not discontinue abruptly at some defined place, as for example at 2 hours per week of exercise. Yet the research tells us and tells us emphatically that doing more than 18-20 minutes per day of walking will produce little added benefit to our health. This contradicts nearly all public recommendations about exercise.

This finding puts another arrow into the heart of that calorie theory of exercise and health. It shows again that very large numbers of added calories of exercise will not necessarily produce more benefits to health. What process or mechanism could explain such an unexpected result?

This leads us directly to my new Heart Theory of Exercise and Cardiofitness that upsets much past thinking about what kinds of exercise are really useful. And the Heart Theory explains easily why a limit to cardiofitness benefits from exercise duration is not only likely but expectable. It seems to explain the results of nearly all of the research we have. More on this follows.

The key mechanism by which exercise protects from heart disease is improved cardiofitness. Thus an important question becomes, "Does cardiofitness also stop improving after two hours of exercise is done?" If so, then this explains why the risk of heart disease stops improving from walking after two hours a week. The following chapter shows that more than two hours of any exercise per week at a given intensity also does not improve cardiofitness usefully. This is the core reason why risk of heart disease is not usefully reduced by exercise of more than two hours per week. I leave this here with what now appears to be a well-confirmed truth:

There is no useful research evidence now available that shows that aerobic exercise of more that 2 hours per week at a given intensity will usefully reduce further the risk of heart disease for healthy persons.

This does not mean that exercising more than this 2 hours will produce zero benefit. There should be some small benefits for reducing weight for the obese. Diabetics will obtain further benefit. There may be as discussed later a small further benefit to cholesterol and other factors. But I will show that the benefits of these other factors are small and contribute perhaps about one-sixth of the benefits of cardiofitness. Except for results on diabetics, these effects on risk of heart disease were too small to be measured even by the very largest research studies now done.

Why Didn't the Researchers Find This Two-Hour Limit?

Most individual researchers did note that the effect of walking pace was larger and more significant than was the effect of walking duration. In fact, a recently-published meta-analysis found a much lesser and less significant effect on risk of heart disease for exercise duration than for intensity. But the idea that there is a time limiting benefit for exercise duration would have been considered improbable.

It was only when this first global analysis brought the results of all studies into similar view that the surprising effect was discovered. Global analysis frequently reveals findings from multiple research results that could not be observed from any individual study or from a usual statistical meta-analysis that develops only an average overall risk.

Benefits for Reducing Risk of Heart Disease by Walking Are Well Established.

The above studies verify that walking reduces risk of heart disease. But the serious question is, "How and how long and how fast do we need to walk to substantially reduce this unwanted risk?"

We do have an accurate effect of walking pace from the results of most of the available studies. We also can derive a useful effect of walking duration for the first two hours per week of walking from most of the study results.

Table 2-2

Table 2-2	Risk Reductions in Heart Disease for Walking at Different Paces and Durations						
Walking Pace Miles per Hour	1.5	2.0	2.5	3.0	3.5	4.0	4.5
Walking Duration Minutes per Week							
30 minutes	1.04	1.06	1.10	1.14	1.16	1.19	1.23
60 minutes	1.06	1.14	1.20	1.30	1.35	1.43	1.51
90 minutes	1.08	1.19	1.30	1.45	1.56	1.72	1.85
120 minutes or more	1.11	1.25	1.41	1.61	1.79	2.04	2.27

Table 2-2 shows how walking pace and duration reduce risk of heart disease. Look first at the bottom row of values that show how increasing walking pace reduces the risk of heart disease for the maximum beneficial exercise time of two hours each week. As before, higher values are better. Reduction in risk is only 1.11 times for a stroll at 1.5 miles per hour. Reduction in risk from walking moves up to 1.41 times or to a 4 times more benefit for an average walking pace of 2.5 miles per hour, to 1.79 times for walking at a quite brisk 3.5 miles per hour, and to a much higher 2.27 times for walking at a fast 4.5 miles per hour. And benefits do increase as expected with duration of exercise done up to two hours each week.

This research clearly endorses the statement "Walking is good for health." But this generality may not mean much. Walking at a slow speed produces so little benefit to normal healthy people that it is close to useless. Our health benefit from walking depends substantially on how fast we walk. It has been estimated that typical mall walking may be at a pace of 2.5 miles per hour. Brisk walking may be at rates of 3 and 3.5 miles per hour. Very few people walk at a regular pace of 4 miles per hour or higher.

Walking for health even at the now confirmed maximum of 2 hours per week still takes substantial time. As a walker you want to make that time spent as useful and possible to your health. A first question of interest is, "How fast do you now walk?" I discuss in Chapter 15 various ways for measuring your walking distance and pace. Without this knowledge about walking pace you probably would continue to walk at the usual pace.

A most practical approach will be to just keep trying to walk a bit faster than usual, and maintain this gradually faster pace. After time you almost certainly will become comfortable when walking faster.

People need to understand clearly the importance to their health of their walking pace. The word 'brisk' in a recommendation can mean very little. People need to actually measure how fast they walk. A potentially better alternative is to measure exercise heart rates during walking. The real key to cardiofitness is exercise of the heart. Much more on this follows later.

How a Walking Program Can Be of Little Value for Health

The two hour per week maximum of exercise that the heart muscle can utilize creates another problem in designing an exercise program Suppose you walk aerobically to or during a job for say a half hour each day. Done a usual 5 times a week, this develops more than the needed two hours of walking. Now if you add to this an exercise program of more walking around the neighborhood during your leisure time, you probably will be wasting a lot of time. You will be doing more than the two hours of exercise that is most useful for health.

This tells you that for obtaining further exercise benefits you must do your leisure time exercise at a significantly higher intensity than that obtained from your usual walking to or on a job. You will not gain more cardio benefit by doing any kind of cardio exercise at an intensity similar to that done in your usual walking.

How Much Exercise Do We Need?

A key problem with much advice about exercise for health is a lack of any perspective about how much exercise is needed. Research studies really show mostly that exercise is "good to do." Any exercise is "good." This may have led to the absurd advice that "All we need to do is to do some walking. There is no purpose in doing that high intensity exercise."

This is wrong. There is no such thing as a single program for exercise that is best for everyone. I will show that we can develop far more health benefit by doing more intensive exercise. Your benefits can change from near zero to extremely high, depending on how intensively and consistently you exercise. But there must be some balance between time and energy spent and benefits to our health. This is a personal problem that requires a decision to be made by each of us.

I propose in this book two goals for improving health. A first goal is an improvement in cardiofitness of 10%. The second, or good goal, is an improvement in cardiofitness of 20%. These goals are for improvement above the cardiofitness level of those that do limited exercise now. Each improvement of 1 unit or 1% in cardiofitness reduces risk of heart disease by 6.4%. As before, the first goal thus develops a reduction in risk of heart disease by 1.85 times. The second goal requires a reduction in risk of 3.5 times. If the first goal is maintained during life it will on average increase likely years of healthful days of life by 3 to 3½ years. Maintaining the second goal could add about 7 years of healthy days to an average life.

Why consider these specific goals? The first goal of 10% is one that I feel nearly every now healthy person should be able to develop as part of responsible personal self-care. It can be obtained by walking at a bit over 3.5 miles per hour for 2 hours each week, or from easy to do exercise programs I will discuss. If done at the national level, the number of US heart attacks by 1.85 times could provide a major contribution to the public health.

The second goal of 20% is more challenging, but should be obtainable from convenient monitored exercise of two hours each week. This should be a goal for any health-interested person. It usually will require somewhat more intensive exercise than walking, but it still usually can be developed from moderate exercise.

These goals are arbitrary, and you may wish to adopt lower or even much higher goals. But we need benchmarks like these to provide a perspective of the potential benefits . Most men and women who develop either of these 10% or 20% exercise goals at middle age should able to maintain these goals as they move into older and even to oldest ages.

The Heart Theory of Exercise Suggests What Happens

This Heart Theory, which is described in more detail in chapters following and in Appendix 5, explains much of what has been very puzzling about the research on exercise. As before, it also upsets many past ideas about how exercise develops health benefits.

Our cardiovascular system is in part of muscle. Cardiofitness is a measure of a physical capability that determines how effectively our heart can circulate blood and its nutrients throughout its extensive system of arteries, veins and capillaries. The Heart Theory holds that cardiofitness develops from the building of heart muscle by the same process that strengthens other body muscles such as those in arms and legs. This concept is not new. What is new is the specific way that cardiofitness develops – or will not develop usefully - from different kinds of exercise. A higher blood flow developed throughout the cardiovascular system provides a higher exercise intensity similar to that produced by the lifting of more weight in a weightlifting program. Muscle builds from the added blood flow in the cardio system and duration of this higher blood flow. Muscle builds similarly from the weight size and number of repetitions of lifting it in a resistance exercise program.

Physical strength develops from high-intensity exercise for some useful time each week. Cardiofitness tends to develop similarly from the highest intensity of heart and cardiovascular exercise maintained for two hours per week. Heart and cardiovascular exercise produced by higher than usual flows of blood both strengthens the heart muscle and enlarges cardio blood vessels and keeps them more open.

There are limits to the rate at which muscles can improve in capability. You can increase strength from weightlifting only gradually. More than 3 sessions of lifting a given weight a useful number of repetitions per week usually will accomplish no further benefit. In order to increase strength you have move steadily to larger weights.

Cardiovascular muscle acts in the same way. Doing more than about two hours of this cardiovascular exercise each week at the same intensity cannot improve the cardiovascular system any faster. More about this is in Appendix 3 and Appendix 5.

Some Observations about Walking Pace

My wife and I have enjoyed many cruises. They provide a fascinating opportunity to watch people walk, either on the promenade deck that provides for general walking around the entire ship or on the smaller exercise track usual on a top deck. The number of laps per mile usually is shown. A dozen serious walkers on the top deck in the morning before breakfast on our most recent cruise were averaging 4.5 mph. I was doing my maximum rate of 4.7 mph (at two to three times the age of the others) and two fit younger women passed me probably going about 5 mph.

Later in the day many dozens of the ship population were walking around the wide promenade deck. At 4.7 mph I was racing past nearly all of the men and women walking there then. Many and probably most were not walking fast enough to improve their health very much. It seems unlikely that these people ever heard the message about the benefits of walking faster.

CHAPTER 3

Cardio Exercise and Cardiofitness

We have excellent research on the health benefits of walking that show how much you need to walk to obtain useful health benefits. In contrast, very little direct research exists on the health benefits of jogging, running, swimming, or other exercise such as using the treadmill or pedaling an exercise bicycle.

A host of unanswered questions exist. How much health benefit comes from jogging, running, or swimming? Is this benefit vs. walking small or large? How long and fast do we need to swim or run for benefit? How does benefit from resistance exercise or calisthenics compare with that from say running? Can we get more cardiofitness and health benefit by walking on a treadmill or using an exercise bicycle? Does the two hour per week limit for effectiveness of exercise on risk of disease apply to all exercise or just to walking?

Fortunately, we do not need direct research on each of these other kinds of exercise to answer these questions. We have an abundance of research that demonstrates the importance of cardiofitness on risk of heart and other diseases as measured by VO2 Max and the CFR. We also have a treasure trove of physiology research that shows the cardiofitness benefits in VO2 Max and CFR for doing nearly any kind and/or amount of aerobic-type exercise. Thus we can merge these two different families of research to learn how any kind of exercise can change cardiofitness, and how this change will translate to risk of disease.

27

Incredibly, much of this important physiology research on how exercise can improve cardiofitness has received little publicity and has not been used effectively. Some of this research focused on how exercise improved risk factors such as cholesterol, triglycerides and blood pressure. Although these risk factors are improved by exercise, they provide only a tiny fraction of the overall health benefit of cardiofitness. More on this follows in Chapter 7.

Cardio Exercise:
From Physiology to Cardiofitness to Health. The Key Is the CFR

The physiology research studies involved carefully designed and monitored amounts of exercise for groups of men and women who exercised from 10 weeks to a year. The Life Ahead paper, which includes the scientific analysis of this research, provides a comprehensive listing of 75 different exercise results from 30 of the more useful of these studies.[29] Results from these studies were expressed as percentage improvements in VO2 that are the same as percentage improvements in CFR. The risks found in epidemiology studies as in Table 1-1 all were compared similarly with the CFR differences of their participants.

The research noted in Chapter 1 shows that each unit increase in cardiofitness of one CFR unit decreases the risk of heart disease by 6.4%. Thus with a common basis for the epidemiology and physiology research we can estimate the probable change in risk of heart disease for any change in CFR produced by exercise.

Good Cardio Exercise Produces Impressive
Cardiofitness and Likely Health Benefits

The question needing an answer is, "How did the improvements in cardiofitness obtained by those that exercised in exercise programs compare with the differences in cardiofitness that were related to risks of heart disease?" Please look at Table 3-1 that shows how cardiofitness improved in eleven different exercise studies that involved vigorous exercise. The men and women in these various programs usually participated for periods of about 24 weeks.

The important results in Table 3-1 are those in Column 5 for the improvements in cardiofitness as CFR obtained by those that exercised. Improvements ranged from 20 to 47 CFR with usual value of about 25. Column 6 shows that calculated improvement in risk of heart disease av-

Table 3-1

Table 3-1.
Good Cardio Exercise can Produce Excellent Improvements in Cardiofitness, and More Years of Healthy Days of Life

1	2	3	4	5	6	7	8
Sex	Age	Exercise hrs/week	Exercise Heart Rate	Increase in CFR	Risk ratio	Added years of Health Life	Type of Exercise
W	30	3	141	20	3.6	6.8	Walking at 5 mph
M	49	2.7	140	25	5.0	8.6	Walking at 4.7 mph
M	47	1.5	150	23	4.4	7.8	Running
M	46	2	135	25	5.0	8.6	Heart rate monitored exercises
M	27	2	159	27	5.6	9.2	Exercise bicycle high intensity 12 week program only
M	65	2	145	26	5.3	8.8	Same as above on older group
M	64	2.9	143	24	4.6	8.3	Various, walking, running, bicycle
W	64	3.1	139	21	3.8	7.2	Same as above for women
M	47	2.2	154	47	10+	10+	High cholesterol men, cycling
M	42	1.7	158	22	4.1	7.5	Cycling to monitored calories
MW	48	1.5	141	28	6.0	9.5	Heart rate treadmill walking

eraging more than 5 times. If maintained, these risk changes translate into from 7.2 to 10+ more years of healthy life as in column 7.

This confirms that good cardio exercise has the potential for developing most of the important reductions in risk of heart disease found from the epidemiology studies. These results usually were for exercising about a half year. Benefits should improve about 20-25% further for a full year of this exercise.

I have suggested a first goal improvement in cardiofitness of 10% and a good improvement goal of 20%. Table 3-1 shows that the good level of 20 or 20% improvement was actually met or exceeded by these eleven actual monitored exercise programs on both men and women. Even those that performed very fast walking at or near 5 miles per hour, as in the first two rows of Table 1, did reach or exceed the desirable 20% good cardiofitness goal.

A problem with the results in Table 3-1 is that actual exercise heart rates listed in column 4 probably were in the range of 140 beats per minute or higher. These are higher exercise heart rates than would be appropriate for the moderate exercise that now is preferred. I will show later how most people can reach the 10% goal and how many can reach the 20% goal from more moderate exercise.

Other fascinating findings emerge from this treasure trove of physiology research. The same improvements in cardiofitness were obtained by women as were obtained by men. The studies produced similarly improved risk ratios and health benefits for adults at ages from 27 to 85. Usual times of exercise were about two hours per week. But as a usual disappointment, no useful improvements in the CFR of cardiofitness were obtained in this research for either calisthenics or resistance exercise. More on this follows.

That Puzzling 2-Hour Limit for Exercise Benefits Is Confirmed Again!

Research on walking showed that only two hours per week of a given exercise intensity was effective in reducing risk of heart disease. Cardiofitness is the primary exercise factor that relates accurately to risk of heart disease. This implied that cardiofitness also might not be improved by more than this same two hours per week of exercise.

I searched for any and all evidence supporting or denying this. My finding is: Exercise of a given intensity of more than two hours per week produces no further improvement in cardiofitness. This is the core reason why exercise of more than this two hours produced little if any further reduction in risk of heart disease.

A study by Ready[34] tested similar groups of women that walked the same hour long program 3 and 5 days per week. The 3-day group gained 12 in CFR; the 5-day group gained only a similar 13 CFR. If benefits had continued as usually expected after two hours of exercise, the 5-day group should have obtained an improvement of 20 CFR.

A large study of 350 persons by Hellerstein found that those who trained about 1½ hours per week did better than those training ¾ hour per week. But those training about 2½ hours per week obtained no further benefit over those training 1½ hours[35]

Each of these studies verified that no further cardiofitness benefits were obtained for exercise times more than two hours per week. I could not find more direct comparisons like these for durations of cardio exercise of less and more than two hours per week at the same intensity. But the database in the scientific paper includes 75 comparisons of changes in cardiofitness developed from different kinds, amounts, and durations of exercise.[29] I set up a model to test from this substantial database how various exercise durations improved cardiofitness. As was done for the research data on heart disease, the results on development of cardiofitness were organized in order of exercise hours per week.

The Conclusion: Aerobic Exercise Duration to only 2 Hours per Week Improves Cardiofitness

More about this and other evidence supporting this 2 hour per week limit for exercise effectiveness is shown in Appendix 3.

Thus we have this surprising and even shocking two hour per week limit for effective aerobic exercise confirmed from two entirely different sets of research. The research on walking and heart disease showed no further effect of walking beyond two hours per week in reducing risk of heart disease. This was from results of nine different studies that included some of the largest and most respected-yet sets of epidemiology research.

The research on 75 different cardio exercise amounts also shows that cardiofitness also is not improved usefully from exercise of more than two hours a week. A very large and important study reviewed in Appendix 3 also found no benefit for more than two hours per week of exercise on risk of death from all causes.

The research on cardiofitness included results for all types of exercise. Thus it appears that the two hour limit of effectiveness of exercise applies not just for walking but for all kinds of aerobic exercise. Cardio system muscle simply will improve at its own rate, and can't be forced to improve faster from more exercise. As mentioned before, this same thing happens in other resistance exercise.

Intensity vs. Calories of Exercise

The theory that the benefits of exercise are related directly to the calories of physical activity usually assumes that exercise duration and intensity are the same and interchangeable. It assumes that we can exercise for a longer time at a low intensity and gain the same benefit as exercising at a higher intensity for a shorter time. This is the theory that has led to the arguably incorrect recommendations that people should walk 30 or 60 minutes every day.

Fifty years of physiological and epidemiological research has shown that this is false. There is no useful relationship between calories of exercise and risk of major disease. As I explained before, the Cooper Institute Group found five times the reduction in risk of heart disease for fewer cardiofitness calories than Paffenbarger found for ordinary physical activity calories. The mail carriers found no more benefit from 15 times more calories than did others that walked far less.

The finding that more than two hours per week of exercise at a given intensity produces no more health or cardio benefit demolishes this calorie or physical activity theory. Despite all of this evidence, some researchers continue to use calories of exercise as a basis for their conclusions.

Physiologists have demolished the calorie theory of exercise further and decisively by direct scientifically-planned experiments. An example by Gary O'Donovan and others divided most of sixty-four previously sedentary men into two exercise groups.[30] For the first 8 weeks each group exercised similarly with gradually increasing amounts of exercise. Starting at 8 weeks the low intensity group continued exercised at a level of 60% of a function of VO2 Max or at about a 130 heart rate for 133 minutes per week. The high intensity group exercised at 80% of the function of VO2 Max or a heart rate of about 150 for a lesser 100 minutes per week. Each group thus exercised *at the same measured calories per week.*

The exercise duration per week of the high intensity group was designed to keep both groups at the same total calories of energy expended. For the first 8 weeks each group as expected obtained similar improvement. But starting immediately at 8 weeks, and at the time the two groups started to exercise at different intensities, the cardiofitness of the high intensity group pulled away from that of the low intensity group.

The cardiofitness of the low intensity group peaked out and reached a plateau at 2.95 ml of oxygen that converts to a CFR of about 96, a 9% gain vs. its initial fitness of 88 CFR. The high intensity group reached an average cardiofitness of 110 CFR vs. a starting value of 90 CFR for a more than twice higher improvement of 22%. A moderately higher intensity level of a given number of exercise calories thus produced more than a twice higher improvement in cardiofitness!

At least three other researchers have found this same thing. Gossard found that cardiofitness increased only 8% in the low intensity vs. 17% in the high intensity group for those exercising the same overall activity calories.[31] Crouse found that cardiofitness increased 26% in quite low fit men exercising at lower intensity but increased 47% for those exercising a shorter time expending the same calories at higher intensity.[32] Krause found that a high intensity exercise group improved 2.5 times more in cardiofitness than did a lower exercise intensity group that exercised the same overall calories.[33]

I will note later that the new Heart Theory explains and forecasts approximately the differences in cardiofitness obtained in these scientifically designed research studies. Thus we now have at least four carefully managed scientifically designed studies of the calorie and exercise intensity controversy. They all found the same thing. Exercise intensity – and not energy calories – is the verified factor that produces cardiofitness.

Cardiofitness Thus Develops Mostly from Exercise Intensity

The anti-fitness advocates who have been demeaning the value of good cardio exercise will not like this conclusion. But let us listen to research, science and reality, not dogma and wishful thinking. Our research now shows overwhelmingly that exercise intensity is primary to the development of both cardiofitness and its improvement of health. We can exercise usefully for up to two hours a week. Beyond this, the attainment of higher cardiofitness will require higher exercise intensity.

But I will show next how we still can protect our health from adequately monitored moderate exercise. We have confirmed research showing that a first goal of 10% increase in cardio benefits can be developed from a quite brisk walking pace of about 3.6 miles per hour. Cardio exercise at higher exercise heart rates for about 2 hours each week can produce 2 to 3 times this benefit. Most people probably can also achieve these higher benefits from moderate exercise. But to accomplish this, exercise must be carefully designed, carried out, and monitored.

The bottom line now is this: Those that want to protect their health need to consider developing a program of good acceptable cardio exercise. This does not have to be very high heart rate exercise. But a really useful exercise program for health does require exercise at a useful exercise intensity. We must develop our aerobic exercise benefits for a duration maximum of 2 hours each week.

How Do We Measure Cardio Exercise Intensity?

We measure our exercise heart rates. Cardiofitness by definition is a physical fitness of the heart and its accompanying cardiovascular system. Cardiofitness is produced by aerobic exercise of the heart. The heart can exercise in only one way: By beating faster than usual. This idea is hardly new. It has been advised and talked about now for at least four decades. Uncounted millions of people have successfully measured their heart rates during exercise programs.

Some experts do not like the idea of measuring heart rates. This controversy may have resulted in the inadequate recommendations about the exercise the public should do starting in 1996. One reason for the opposition to measuring heart rates has been the unfriendly method of specifying exercise heart rates as percentages of a maximum heart rate. Another is the incorrect implication that a measured heart rate meant a high heart rate.

The new Heart Method for developing cardiofitness does not use those troublesome percentages. There is a much easier way that also is more accurate and scientifically valid. It is Heart Rate Elevation and the simple and straightforward direct use of our exercise heart rate. The next chapter tells about this. We can develop goals for cardiofitness from properly monitored moderate heart rates that are very simple to measure and use. This leads us to simple practical exercise programs that individuals can use to keep themselves cardiofit.

CHAPTER 4

GETTING TO ANY DESIRED CARDIOFITNESS AND THE MASTER TABLES.

A next question becomes, "What exercise heart rate do we need to maintain to develop a healthful level of cardiofitness?" The Heart Method holds that cardiofitness develops from exercise of the heart that produces higher rates of blood flow in the cardiovascular system for a particular length of time each week. The pressure developed from the more than usual volume of blood being circulated by the heart is the counterpart of the weight level used in resistance exercise. The heart usually pumps a near equal volume of blood with each stroke after its rate is modestly elevated. Thus the volume of blood being circulated and pressure exerted by this motion depend on the amount of blood being circulated by each beat.

This chapter tells about the two important keys needed to develop a measure of this flow rate of blood that produces our all-important cardiofitness. These are first, Heart Rate Elevation and second, the Master Tables of Cardiofitness. This new technology shows how nearly any desired and achievable level of cardiofitness can be developed from various amounts and different kinds of exercise for those of any age. Heart rate Elevations are simply the exercise heart rate minus the Low Resting Heart Rate.

Although the Master Table approach is simple, if you want things even more simple a following chapter tells about a method that most people can use to develop a useful improvement in cardiofitness without using any tables. I call this program CARDIO 120. I also suggest an easy to use Cardiofitness Point Method for developing the effective cardio exercise you need to do to reach either a first goal or a good goal for cardiofitness improvement.

But you should learn about and measure your Low Resting Heart Rate, as described following, in order to understand how the Heart Method works. This is an important number needed to manage your cardiofitness effectively.

The Low Resting Heart Rate

Our heart usually beats at its lowest rate in the morning before breakfast and before doing any exercise. This lowest heart rate is called the Low Resting Heart Rate. This lowest resting heart rate supports our basal metabolism, or the energy needed to keep our body warm and alive. This is commonly referred to as an exercise intensity level of one metabolic unit, or 'one met.' Our resting heart rate during the day usually will be 5-10 beats per minute above this lowest rate due to energy demands of food digestion and daily physical tasks.

The Low Resting Heart Rate is a marker of the zero level of our exercise. An average person of 150 pounds burns about a hundred calories per hour and this requires the heart to beat at about 70 beats per minute at the heart's usual lowest level during a day. This energy is needed just to keep us alive and warm. It is not a part of our exercise.

As we do any kind of physical activity our heart rate will move above this low resting rate. The level of our exercise determines how much our heart rate increases above its low resting rate. We call this difference between an exercise heart rate and the low resting heart rate the Heart Rate Elevation. When we are exercising usefully, nearly all of the elevation in our exercise heart rate above our resting heart rate will be directly due to our exercise. It is first useful to understand more about our low resting heart rate.

I show in Figure 4-1 a diagram of how a man's resting heart rate varied during a day. His lowest rate was about 75 beats per minute in the morning before breakfast. This is his Low Resting Heart Rate.

After breakfast his resting heart rate increased steadily about 12 beats per minute higher about an hour and a half later. Then it moved back down again until it was near its low resting rate again just before lunch. The same thing happened after lunch and after dinner. His smoothed resting heart rate moved up to supply the energy for food digestion, and then moved

Figure 4-1

Resting Heart Rate before and after Meals and Exercise

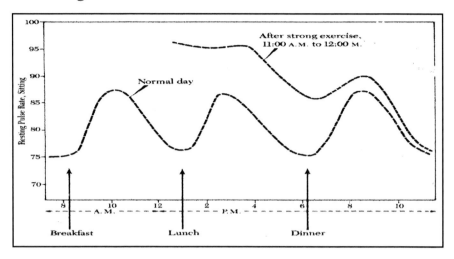

down after this process was mostly completed.

Figure 4-1 shows that a resting heart rate taken at random times during the day can vary up to 10 beats per minute just due to times taken relative to those of meals. Your resting heart rate also can move up for a variety of factors such as nervousness or anxiety. This is the reason that it is so important to self measure your low resting heart rate before breakfast, after fasting during the night, before any food is taken, and after sitting quietly for two minutes or more.

The upper line shows this man's resting heart rates taken after 45 minutes of vigorous aerobic exercise just before noon. His resting rate soon after his exercise was a high 20 beats per minute above the low resting heart rate of 75. This was due to what can be called post-exercise calorie after-burn.

The energy needed to fuel the body's activities comes from two sources. First, short-term energy needs for exercise are supplied from glycogen stores in the body. But if a continuing energy demand is imposed, as from steady walking or running, the heart rate increases sufficiently to directly supply the energy need. This is aerobic exercise.

It usually takes up to about three minutes of steady exercise for the heart rate to increase sufficiently to fully supply this energy need. During this time part of the energy of continuing exercise is supplied from glycogen stores in the body. Also, there may be some smaller drawdown of glycogen during aerobic exercise. After exercise is stopped, the heart will beat faster than usual for up to 12 or more hours to replace its desired reserve of glycogen. You can see from upper line in Figure 4-1 how resting heart rate continued at a higher than usual rate and then gradually moved down to a more usual level as these glycogen stores were replaced.

This shows that exercise calories measured during the time of actual exercise do not include all of the calorie burn of the exercise. Any fairly intensive aerobic exercise should create some anaerobic debt that will produce this calorie after-burn. The anaerobic debt from resistance type exercise and its after-burn can be larger than that from aerobic exercise because most energy for this type of exercise is provided from body glycogen stores.

This demonstrates further why a low resting heart rate must be taken after a night's fast and before any exercise is done. Usual resting heart rates taken in a doctor's office or in an exercise program can be 5 to 15 beats per minute higher than a true low resting heart rate. You also can be a bit nervous when the resting rate is taken by a doctor or other health professional. Thus to obtain an accurate measure of your heart rate at a true metabolic level you should take this heart rate by yourself. You may be able to get a useful low resting heart rate just before a noon or evening meal if you have not exercised and have not eaten any intervening food or snacks.

Some individuals have atypical resting heart rates. This can be due to heart problems, as for example irregular or skipped beats. Medications can cause heart rates to be lower or higher than usual. Some people can have genetic differences in the way their hearts beats. I do not have any good solution for those with such problems. But if your health is good and you are medically approved for exercise, I suggest you just take some average number, as for example a value from Table 4-1, or just assume a usual value of 70. The Heart Theory Method will still be useful. You do not need to know your low resting heart rate to develop a CARDIO 120 program.

Reductions in your low resting heart rate can be welcome and even exciting. This can provide a simple in-body measurement that shows how your cardiofitness is improving. By taking your heart rate carefully at various times during the day you also can gain an understanding of how energy in your body is changing.

Low Resting Heart Rates and Cardiofitness

As our cardiofitness improves, our low resting heart rates usually will decline. This is due to the fact that our heart becomes more capable of pumping blood as it is exercised in the same way arms are strengthened from their exercise. As our heart becomes more capable it requires fewer beats per minute to supply our needs for basal metabolism.

Table 4-1

Usual Low Resting Heart Rates and Cardiofitness					
Usual Life Style	Low Resting Heart Rate				Cardiofitness in CFR
	Men		Women		
	Minute	10 Sec	Minute	10 Sec	
Mostly Sit and Drive	70+	12	72+	12	90 or lower
Avg Sedentary, little Exercise	65-69	11	68-72	12	89-103
Moderately Active, Some Exercise	60-64	10	63-67	11	104-120
Good Regular Cardio Exercise	55-59	9	58-62	10	121-135
Excellent Regular Aerobic Exercise	48-54	8	52-57	9	136-150

Table 4-1 summarizes results of various studies that showed how low resting heart rates usually decline as cardiofitness improves. I show the low resting heart rates per minute and the rates in 10 seconds that are commonly reported from many exercise programs. The right column shows usual values of the CFR measure of cardiofitness that I have used before and will discuss more following. A value of 100 CFR identifies an average level of cardiofitness for age and gender.

Some people with heart problems have very low or variable heart rates and may even need a pacemaker to keep the rate up. The relationships in Table 4-1 and the technology that follows will not be useful for such individuals. This is a problem needing a doctor's care, and the exercise of anyone with a medical problem such as this should be prescribed by the doctor. All suggestions for exercise made in this book about exercise assume that individuals are initially healthy and medically approved to do exercise. The values for low resting heart rates much below 65-70 in Table 4-1 and in Appendix 1 are for average healthy people with normal heart rate function that do substantial exercise and are cardiofit.

About Heart Rate Elevation

Heart Rate Elevation or the increase in its beating rate above its low resting heart rate is the BIG THING that improves cardiofitness. This elevation identifies an intensity of heart exercise. And it also determines the added amount of blood the heart is pumping when exercising versus the more usual flow at rest. This Heart Rate Elevation added to the low resting heart rate results in an exercise heart rate. Forget for the moment anything you have heard about exercising at some percentage of heart rate. I will explain later that a percentage of maximum rate is not useful for estimating how our cardiofitness will improve.

Our exercise heart rate is the rate we need to monitor during our exercise. But exercise heart rate is not the key number that produces cardiofitness. An athlete with a resting heart rate of a low 40 beats per minute will obtain a large increase in blood flow and strong cardiovascular exercise at a twice higher exercise heart rate of only 80 beats per minute. A sedentary man having an 80 low resting heart rate may need to move up to a 160 heart rate to achieve a similar percentage increase in blood flow. Thus an exercise heart rate per se will not measure the energy or blood flow developed by those having differences in cardiofitness. The amount of blood flow will depend on the product of heart rate elevation and the amount of blood pumped with each beat.

The Effect of Exercise Heart Rate Elevations on Cardiofitness

What exercise heart rate elevation do we need to use when exercising at this two hours in order to reach a cardiofitness level that will produce a good improvement in health? We have an excellent database of 75 comparisons that I described earlier to answer this. This database includes groups that increased their cardiofitness from near zero to 47%, multiple results on groups of both men and women, results for adults of all ages, results for differing exercise durations, and results for times of exercise done from 4 to 50 months.

I extensively tested the accuracy of different methods for measuring how cardiofitness developed from various measures of exercise intensity. The simple exercise heart rate elevation forecast cardiofitness improvement better than did any other method. These included percentages of maximum heart rate and a more involved method known as percentage of VO2 Max that is now used by most researchers. A still better relationship was found between a 1.6 power function of exercise heart rate elevation and development of cardiofitness. This power function is consistent with what would be expected about the energy needed to produce different blood flow rates from chemical engineering. The formulas for the mathematical model that resulted from this analysis and more on how it was developed are provided in Appendix 1 for those interested.

Any inclusion of a maximum heart rate value in a formula for exercise intensity resulted in inaccurate valuations of cardiofitness development for people of different ages. This is because people of all ages develop cardiofitness similarly from a given elevation in heart rate. More on this follows here and is also included in Appendix 4.

This higher power effect of heart rate on cardiofitness also explains in part why walking or running pace can be much more important to risk of heart disease than is walking duration. Walking at 2.5 mph develops 85 units of energy per hour above simply sitting. For walking at 4.5 mph the energy exercising the heart increases to 280 units. Now go to jogging at 6 mph. The heart exercise energy moves up to 500 units per hour.

The Master Tables

I call a relationship between heart rate elevations and time of exercise and cardiofitness development a Master Table. Table 4-2 is the Master Table developed for an average low resting heart rate of 70 beats per minute. By showing tables for different low resting heart rates we can show both the heart rate elevation needed and the exercise heart rates needed for each result. This makes the monitoring of exercise more convenient because exercise heart rates are the actual rates we need to develop during our exercise.

The upper row of numbers in Table 4-2 shows that exercise that produces only a 90 exercise heart rate will produce for this person only a 2 or 2% improvement in CFR after a year of this exercise. If exercise heart rate is moved up to 100, the benefit will go three times higher 6 CFR. An increase in exercise heart rate to 110 beats per minute will increase benefit 50% to 9 in CFR. These estimates are all for two hours per week of this exercise done by an average sedentary man or woman.

The Master Table provides something I feel is both new and important. We can learn how our simple exercise heart rate produces our cardiofitness and health benefits. Previous recommendations about exercise heart rates at percentages of maximum heart rate could be difficult to understand and use, and do not explain accurately how cardiofitness develops from exercise.

Table 4.2

Cardiofitness Improvement in CFR from Exercise Heart Rates over one Year Resting Heart Rate = 70		
Elevation above Low Resting Rate	Exercise Heart Rate	Improvement in CFR from a Starting Level of 90 CFR Two hours/week of exercise
20	90	2
30	100	6
40	110	9
50	120	13
60	130	18
70	140	23
80	150	29
90	160	34

Note the importance of exercise heart rate and heart rate elevation to the development of cardiofitness. A difference of just 10 beats per minute in exercise heart rate can mean a difference of 50% in the CFR improvement obtained. Many people have done their cardio exercise at all kinds of unknown or varying heart rates. This can be very inefficient.

An important finding from this Master Table is that exercise at a moderate 120 beats per minutes can produce a useful 13% cardio improvement for a man or woman having a 70 low resting heart rate. But this benefit can be mostly lost if exercise heart rates drop to 100 beats per minute or less. This 13% improvement is better than the 10% suggested for a first goal for cardiofitness.

Let's try an example using Table 4-2. Suppose a man has this low resting heart rate of about 70 and now does very little cardio type exercise. His CFR, or cardiofitness level, probably will be in the range of 90. He would like to reach a first goal of an improvement of 10 CFR or 10% in cardiofitness.

Table 4-2 shows that an elevation of 40 beats per minute (in the left column) above the resting rate of 70 would produce an actual exercise heart rate of 110 (in the middle column). At a 110 exercise heart rate, the value in Table 4-2 for 2 hours or more of exercise is 9 CFR (in the right column). This tells us that if he exercised two hours a week at a heart rate of 110 for one year, his predicted increase in CFR would be 9 .

Similarly, a 120 heart rate would improve CFR by 13 . Interpolation suggests he should target an exercise heart rate a bit above 110 or about 112 to reach a goal of a 10% improvement in CFR. If continually maintained during life, this improvement in cardiofitness could add an average of 3½ healthy years. As shown in Appendix 1, about 75-80% of this cardiofitness should develop in a half year of exercise.

You might wish to select different targets than the 10 CFR for a first and 20 CFR for the good goal that I suggest. As example, suppose you find exercising at a 120 heart rate is comfortable and you are medically approved for and have been accustomed to exercising at this rate. You can choose to target the improvement of 13 CFR listed in Table 4-2 for a 120 heart rate program. Or you can use a still higher exercise heart rate if this is comfortable.

Appendix 1 includes four Master Tables for low resting heart rates of 50, 60, 70, and 80 beats per minute. Also included are the factors to these values for exercise durations of less than 2 hours per week, for times of exercise less than a year, and other factors. I have placed these important tables at this position in the book so that you can find them easily.

How does this help us? Without the Master Tables most of us really are exercising in the dark. We have no idea how useful our exercise is. Suppose you were walking, your low resting rate was 70 and your exercise heart rate was measured at 90. You can see from Table 4-2 that this would produce only a trivial improvement of 2 in CFR after a full year of walking. This would produce little improvement in health.

Millions of people today are faithfully walking 30 minutes every day like this with the misguided understanding that they are "getting their proper exercise." They are mostly wasting a monumental amount of time obtaining only a fraction of the health benefit they could be achieving.

Exercise Heart Rates Need to Be Measured Carefully for Gains in Cardiofitness.

This new technology shows that accurate exercise heart rates are of key importance. Consider some results from Table 4.2. Walking at a 90 exercise heart rate in the previous paragraph would produce an improvement in CFR of only 2. Move that exercise heart rate to 110 from quite brisk walking, and the improvement will be 9 or 9%, a far larger gain. Move the exercise rate to just 10 more or 120 beats per minute, and gain will be 13 CFR.

Present official recommendations about exercise attempt to identify exercise intensity without measuring heart rates. This approach can identify widely varying levels of actual heart rate and true exercise intensity. These variations can include exercise heart rates that are nearly useless for developing health benefits or too high for needed or even prudent exercise. There has been inadequate understanding by experts and researchers of the key importance of accurately measured and maintained heart rates in developing cardiofitness.

Another factor that has been poorly recognized is the importance of resting heart rate and heart rate elevation. It is the *elevation in heart rate* above its low resting or metabolic rate that adds blood flow and develops cardiofitness. A 100 exercise heart rate identifies a 50 elevation for one with a 50 resting heart rate. This seemingly modest exercise heart rate for two hours a week from a 50 resting rate will produce a near good goal improvement of 19% in CFR. This same exercise heart rate for one with a 70 resting heart rate will produce only an inadequate 6% gain. The added blood flow rate that produces cardiofitness is almost directly proportional to heart rate elevation above its resting rate.

Using the Master Tables for Those Now Exercising

The Master Tables also can provide an interesting guide for those that are now exercising. Suppose as a young enthusiast with a 70 resting heart rate you are running 3 miles a day six days a week at a 150 heart rate. 18 miles a week at say about 8 miles per hour would put you at more than the 2 hours of duration needed for maximum benefits. Table 4-2 shows that at a 150 average exercise heart rate, you probably are either producing or moving toward a fine 29 improvement in CFR. You thus should be achieving much more than my good goal of and improvement of 20% improvement in cardiofitness.

You now have a basis for assessing what you probably are achieving and for reassessing what you wish to do. A first suggestion would be to cut back to the two hours a week maximum time for useful exercise. You could reduce your intensity to a heart rate of 140 or 135 and still obtain a quite useful improvement in cardiofitness. But with this exercise your resting heart rate should be much below 70, and a new scenario develops at this lower resting rate. In fact, with your running you probably will be obtaining much more that that 29 improvement in CFR at that 150 exercise heart rate. I will discuss more about this later.

A Master Table is a universal table for cardiofitness development from any kind of aerobic type exercise for men and women of any age for one value of low resting heart rate. The heart does not know or care what physical exercise is producing an energy demand. It only knows that it must beat faster at some required heart rate to support this demand.

This faster beating produces the increased blood flow that provides its exercise. The Master Table values represent average results for the thousands of individuals that exercised in different programs. Some probably will obtain lower and others higher value results than those in the tables. We have age differences, height differences, weight difference, gender differences and genetic differences in our population. But the present tables should provide a useful first guide for nearly everyone.

Percentage of Maximum Heart Rate is Not Accurate or Useful for Planning Exercise Intensity

The maximum heart rate concept was proposed more than 4 decades ago as a guide to heart rates that were appropriate for exercise by those of differing ages. A percentage of this maximum as for example 85% or 90% provides a useful guide as the highest heart rates we should develop. This use of the maximum heart rate still remains an important guide.

A problem starts, however, when people are asked to exercise at other percentages of this maximum rate, as for example, 50%, 60% and 70%. These levels of heart rate become very inaccurate as a measure of exercise intensity. As example, for 50% of a usually estimated maximum heart rate, an exercise heart rate becomes 85 beats per minute for a 50 year old and 70 beats per minute for an 80 year old. These are useless and incorrect exercise heart rates. At 60% of maximum the heart rates become 102 for a 50 year old and 84 for the 80 year old respectively, still inadequate exercise heart rates for most people. More about the problems and errors involved with use of the maximum heart rate method in estimating exercise intensity is in Appendix 4

Although percentages of maximum heart rate are not used for intensity in the Heart Method, exercise heart rates always should be kept at or below usual safe limits for age. Appendix 4 shows values for 90% of a best formula for maximum heart rates. Exercising at 90% of maximum heart rate is consistent with guides of the American College of Sports Medicine for healthy fit adults. These maximum values suggest maximum exercise

45

heart rates declining from 167 at age 30 to 155 at age 50 and to 136 beats per minute at age 80 and are values useful only for those accustomed to very vigorous exercise. Most emphasis in this book is for programs that should involve much lower exercise heart rates than these maximum exercise rates.

The Heart Method Shows How to Exercise for Health Benefit

The heart rates needed to develop cardiofitness are developed in the Master Tables. These values apply to men and women of all ages from 20 to above 80, and probably to above 90. Cardio research now identifies no difference in the development of cardiofitness from a given exercise heart rate for people of different ages

The fact that older people can obtain good improvements in cardiofitness has also been confirmed further by a meta-analysis of 41 studies of exercise on 2,100 men and women over age 60 that showed an average improvement of 16% in cardiofitness.[78] Women probably need to go to a few beats higher heart rate than do men to get to the same cardiofitness, but the research I analyzed does not identify such a difference with useful accuracy.

Resting Heart Rate Is Important.
And Cardio Feedback Can Be a Major Key to Cardiofitness

Table 4-1 showed that typical low resting heart rates dropped substantially from about 70 to 50 as cardiofitness improved from about 90 CFR for no exercise to above 140 CFR for excellent aerobic exercise. Research suggests that our resting heart rate usually will move down about 1 beat per minute for each improvement of 3 in the CFR. That one beat per minute will be too small an amount to measure, but if you achieve that first 10% improvement goal, your cardiofitness probably will have improved by 10 CFR. Your low resting heart rate now should be lower by about 3 beats per minute.

We now move to what I think is one of the most fascinating new things about cardio exercise. It is what I call Cardio Feedback. This can be a bit mind twisting, so please try to stay with me!

Suppose as in Example 1 above the man exercised consistently at the computed exercise heart rate of 112 for a full year. His low resting heart rate from an improvement of 10 in CFR should move down the above 3 beats per minute or from 70 to 67. Now his Heart Rate Elevation at this same exercise heart rate of 112 will move up from the 42 (112 minus70) original level to a value of about 45 (112 minus 67. That sounds like a small increase. Yet this reduction in resting heart rate has increased heart rate elevation when exercising at the same 112 heart rate. This in turn increases his blood flow at a given exercise heart rate by about 12%.

This higher blood flow now will give him a computed improvement of 11 CFR from Table 4-2 vs. the original desired increase of 10 CFR. This will lower his resting heart rate a bit further. And as resting heart rate goes down some more, his Heart Rate Elevation increases again. And as the Heart Rate Elevation increases again, his gain in cardiofitness goes up again by a little more.

These incremental changes produce over time what is called a Feedback Loop. If you keep firmly at that given exercise heart rate, your low resting rate will also keep moving down. This will increase your heart rate elevation and amount of blood being pumped. Thus your cardiofitness should continue to increase. And over long time, cardiofitness can increase much more than that shown in above Table 4-2 for just one year of exercise.

Another thing also happens. As your resting heart rate moves down, your heart will supply the energy for metabolism from fewer beats. Thus at a given exercise heart rate it will pump more blood with each beat. This mechanism adds even further to that feedback loop. There is another way to understand Cardio Feedback from what happened unwittingly to me that follows.

Feedback produces that high level squealing sound that annoys you when people are adjusting a sound system. The global warming researchers are talking about how feedback from the melting of glaciers can accelerate the warming trend. But cardio feedback from our cardio exercise can be very good thing. It was very good to me.

How I Got to Very High Fitness with a Moderate Exercise Heart Rate from Cardio Feedback

You may never have to exercise at high heart rates to become very cardiofit. I have now been exercising for decades and to my knowledge never exercised regularly at a sustained heart rate above 120 beats per minute. At about age 65 and after about ten years of good cardio exercise, a treadmill test measured me at 52.2 VO2 Max that produces a very high CFR of above 150.

I was astounded. This is a cardiofitness level above that of a usual 20 year old and near that of an athlete. I am no athlete and never was one. How could this very high cardiofitness have developed from a moderate exercise heart rate of only 120 beats per minute? My CFR before starting this type of regular exercise was only 103.

Master Table 4-2 shows a one-year gain of only 15 CFR for a 120 heart rate. This would take me from my starting CFR of 103 to 118. How could I have gotten to a much higher CFR of 150 from this rather modest level of exercise heart rate?

Part of the answer is straightforward. My resting heart rate moved down gradually during the years of good exercise from an initial 70 to below 50 beats per minute. I always measured my exercise heart rate. I also measured my low resting rate frequently. For many years I kept my exercise heart rate close to 120 beats per minute when swimming my usual 3 sessions per week of 72 lengths of the 25 yard pool that added up to 3 miles each week. I also did a modest amount of fast walking and jogging. Thus as my resting heart rate moved down, my heart elevation moved up from about 50 to 70 beats per minute at a 120 per minute exercise heart rate.

When exercising at a 70 heart rate elevation I was obtaining 70% more actual blood flow and heart exercise than when exercising initially at a 50 beat per minute elevation. Recall that energy moves up exponentially from higher exercise heart rates. Table 4-2 shows a gain of 23 CFR for a heart rate elevation of 70. This moved my predicted CFR to 126. This is closer, but still does not forecast how I got to such a high 150 CFR.

That second thing noted above happened. When my resting heart rate moved from 70 to 50, my heart had to pump only 50 times to supply my basal metabolism vs. the 70 times needed at the start of my program. Thus my heart probably pumped 70/50 or about 40% more blood and oxygen with each stroke.

After my resting rate moved down to 50, I could not get my heart rate up above 85 beats per minute even when walking at close to a very fast 5 miles per hour or by doing light jogging. I was getting the same blood flow at a heart rate of 85 that I was formerly getting at a 130 heart rate. It is blood flow – and not just heart rate – that produces heart exercise and cardiofitness.

Now when exercising at 120 heart rate I not only was getting a higher heart rate elevation, but was also pumping 40% more blood with each beat of my heart. My effective elevation was 70 times 1.4 or close to 100. An extension of Table 4-2 forecasts about a 40 increase in CFR for 100 heart rate elevation. This now forecasts a 143 CFR for me, in the range of that measured! The mystery is solved. I obtained a very high cardiofitness from exercising many years at a moderate heart rate of 120. I got there unwittingly because of CARDIO FEEDBACK.

The key to obtaining cardio feedback is to keep that exercise heart rate firmly at a given level. Your heart will effectively continue to exercise more and more as your resting heart rate moves down. This change was not perceived as detectible to me when swimming because it happened slowly over long periods of time. I always felt comfortable at the same 120 exercise heart rate.

But the important message about cardio feedback is this: It probably will never develop unless you do firmly maintained heart-rate-monitored exercise. If you do not do this, your exercise heart rate will just decline as your resting rate declines and you will not develop this benefit. General measures of exercise intensity such as the 'moderate' or 'vigorous' now proposed by our health establishment will not develop this very large potential benefit of cardio feedback that should develop from accurate heart rate monitored exercise.

Cardio Feedback may require a number of years of regular exercise for best benefit. I had no record of how my low resting heart rate moved down, but I do recall it was in the range of 60 for quite a while before it finally descended to a bit below 50 beats per minute.

It seems likely that cardio feedback does happen to others. A group of quite cardiofit older women were measured by Warren[37] at an average CFR of 147. The CFR of the highest cardiofit men and women that were mostly doing good cardio exercise in the Cooper Institute study averaged above 140 CFR. It seems very unlikely that all of these persons maintained the very high heart rate elevations of 90 or more beats per minute that would be needed to develop such levels of cardiofitness in a one year time. The computations I made above are from simple and logical engineering that forecasts that this cardio feedback should happen.

The Appendix Master Tables: The four Master Tables for resting heart rates from 50 to 80 beats per minute are guides to plan your cardio exercise. Use the table closest to your own low resting heart rate. They recognize the logical effect of heart rate elevation on cardiofitness. And they also recognize that a more cardiofit heart will pump more blood per stroke than will an unfit heart.

You can use these tables to estimate the heart rate you need during exercise to develop any achievable level of cardiofitness. I suggest again that a first goal of 10% and a good goal of 20% improvement in cardiofitness vs. sedentary can be useful targets for improvement of health. But as I emphasize frequently, if you are now sedentary, plan your exercise to work up slowly and gradually to these targets.

But you don't have to use these Master Tables if they still puzzle you. I describe in the next chapter a very simple exercise method called CARDIO 120 that should, over the long range, improve the cardiofitness of most participants. This requires no use of tables or formulas. And CARDIO 120 should eventually develop cardio feedback if you keep your exercise heart rate firmly on a target.

If you maintain your exercise heart rates faithfully, your low resting heart rate probably will gradually move down and you will have promoted yourself to the use of a Master Table for a lower resting heart rate. You will obtain more actual heart exercise from a given level of exercise heart rate as your resting rate moves down from good cardio exercise. It can be exciting see your low resting heart rate move down. This can be confirmation that your exercise is producing benefits to your health.

But in order to learn how your low resting heart rate moves down, you must take it yourself in the morning before breakfast for a full minute after sitting for a while. You should not accept a resting heart rates measured either by you or by someone else at some other random time.

Some examples of how you can obtain much more benefit from your exercise at a 120 exercise heart rate as your low resting heart rate declines are interesting. Your gain in one year should be 13 CFR at a low resting heart rate of 70 beats per minute. For a low resting heart rate of 60, your gain should move up to 21 CFR. And if you achieve a low resting rate of 50, that gain can be a very high 32 CFR by exercising at that same heart rate of 120 beats per minute. Once your low resting rate moves down to 60, you will able to develop a good goal of 20% improvement in cardiofitness by exercising at a moderate 120 beats per minute. These average figures assume normal or average heart rate function from change in exercise. They do not include any benefits from cardio feedback that should develop over the years.

Again, it does not matter how you obtain those heart rates. It can be from walking, jogging, running, swimming, treadmill exercise, aerobic dancing or any other exercise capable of producing heart rate elevations. The gains in cardiofitness shown at various heart rates are for average persons and these can vary somewhat for individuals.. Chapter 15 tells more about the many kinds of exercise that can produce cardiofitness.

The first hour of exercise develops nearly 60% of what comes from two hours per week. These values all derive from the referenced database and are averages. Cardiofitness improves only at a rate of about 1% per week. It will improve this useful amount from a modest increase in exercise. The rate of CFR improvement per week cannot be usefully increased by using much larger amounts or higher intensities of exercise.

Work up Carefully If You are Not Cardiofit

You should visit your doctor before starting any serious regular exercise, especially if you now sedentary. Then start exercise at levels of exercise heart rate well below this 120 level, and work up slowly and carefully. One basis is to start by measuring your heart rate at your usual brisk walking pace. Then continue to walk faster to move the heart rate up by only 5 more beats per minute for a full month of multiple exercises per week. If you cannot reach the 120 heart rate by walking, move to another stronger exercise. But continue to move your heart rate up only by that 5 beats per minute each month until you reach the 120 exercise heart rate comfortably. An alternate is to move your exercise heart rate up just 1 beat per 10 or 15 seconds. The following chapter describes in detail the steps you take to improve your cardiofitness using either a CARDIO 120 program or a Managed Cardio program.

Heart Rates Must be Measured

I have mentioned repeatedly that a serious error still made by our health establishment is the lack of a useful target for exercise heart rate. Maintaining a carefully identified heart rate has a double advantage. First, it provides some assurance that a real improvement in cardiofitness will result. Second, it provides a measure that keeps heart rates from becoming too high for prudent self-care.

Running or jogging will produce a usefully elevated heart rate for nearly everyone. But most other exercises will not accomplish this unless heart rates are measured. It simply is impossible to know how much of an exercise is needed for benefit if exercise heart rate is not known. As above, the large potential benefits of cardio feedback will not be obtained without careful heart rate monitoring of exercise.

Would those doing resistance exercise be satisfied with weights unmarked as to number of pounds or kilograms? Would they be satisfied to pick an unmarked weight at random for each exercise session? This is what most people are now doing for the exercise of their hearts. They can be using exercise levels that are unmarked weights and have little idea about the effectiveness of what they are doing. They also can be exercising at a heart rate that is unnecessarily high for their present level of cardiofitness.

I mentioned the fallacy that it is not necessary to measure heart rates for moderate exercise. We just have to walk, and that will give us benefits. Realistically, it can be more important to measure walking heart rates than to measure heart rates for more intense exercise. Millions today may be developing an elevation of only 20 beats per minute elevation above low resting rate when walking. Note again from the Master Tables how CFR and health benefits move up from the 20 elevation to a 30 and then a 40 beat per minute elevation. Figure 3-1 showed the significant effect of walking pace on reduction in risk of heart disease. It is very easy to walk at a pace that is mostly wasting time.

Measuring Your Heart Rate

Most monitored cardio exercise programs teach how to obtain heart rates. Most people take the rate by holding fingers gently over the carotid artery in the neck where it beats most solidly. Aerobic dancing participants often take rates for just 10 seconds and use 10 second targets as 20 for an exercise heart rate of 120 beats per minute. I prefer taking it for 15 seconds and then doubling twice to get the rate. You can take it exercising or can stop exercise and take it immediately for 10 or 15 seconds and still get a pretty good rate.

Measuring exercise heart rates will be very familiar to anyone that has participated in an exercise program such as aerobic dancing or to the many women that have participated in Curves. Measuring a heart rate becomes very simple with practice. Be sure to start your rate count with zero and not at one. Many forget to do this

Treadmills often have devices that measure heart rate directly, but be sure you get a rate that is remains steady and changes only gradually. These rates can fluctuate and be in error. You also can buy heart rate monitors that measure – and more expensive ones that record – rates during an exercise session. The best ones use a strap that fits over your chest. A heart rate monitor can substantially help you in learning of how your heart rates vary during exercise.

Exercising on a quality treadmill that includes a device for measured heart rate can be a near ideal method for developing your cardiofitness. You can set the speed and incline to produce any desired exercise heart rate for a defined time, and watch TV as you exercise.

I discuss next the specific simple exercise programs that can help most people improve their cardiofitness and health both efficiently and effectively.

CHAPTER 5.

Cardio 120 and Managed Cardio

Good cardiofitness can be produced efficiently by exercise done at high heart rates. But moderate exercise is preferred by most of our population. Moderate exercise can be developed more easily and conveniently. Moderate exercise involves less risk of injuries. Exercise is something those of every age should be able to do as they move through the older ages of life. A bias by experts against high heart rate exercise was a key reason for the shift in official exercise recommendations away from what was thought to be high intensity to moderate exercise.

Yet our research shows that we must develop cardiofitness to achieve the major health benefits from exercise. Thus the challenge is to develop effective improvement in cardiofitness from moderate level exercise. A question becomes What is moderate exercise?

Defining moderate exercises as examples such as gardening or walking is not useful. Most gardening time can be spent watering or weeding that hardly is useful aerobic exercise. Walking can vary from near useless to excellent exercise depending on its pace. Developing cardiofitness requires the development of higher than usual maintained cardio flows of blood

The only practical and scientifically useful way to define a level of cardio exercise intensity is by an individual's exercise heart rate. It is exercise of the heart and its cardiovascular system that over time that produces the cardio exercise that benefits health. A typical exercise heart rate for very brisk to fast walking is 110 to 120 beats per minute for most people of all ages. This is the same range of exercise intensity that the Master Tables show is usefully aerobic. Thus it seems reasonable to define 'moderate exercise' as a usual exercise heart rate of 110-120 beats per minute.

Keep in mind that the key factor that moves more blood and that improves cardiofitness is not the exercise heart rate per se but the elevation in this rate above low resting heart rate. If you keep exercising faithfully at 120 beats per minute each week your resting heart rate down and your heart rate elevation will move up. This over time can move your cardiofitness to quite healthful values. This leads to the first suggested cardio exercise program I call CARDIO 120. It simply is this: You exercise two hours each week at an average measured heart rate of between 110 and 120 beats per minute from any selected appropriate exercise. You do not need to use any tables, compute any ratios, or use any formulas. As will follow, you can develop your exercise from any of a wide variety of different exercise methods.

If you prefer and/or have been exercising, you can develop your own guidelines for your exercise with what I call Managed Cardio. This helps you plan exercise to reach objectives for cardiofitness that you can select. I will assume that you have now measured or will measure your low resting heart rate. The further steps needed to develop a CARDIO 120 program follow first.

A Cardio 120 Program

1. First measure your heart rate during exercise. Most people take it best by feeling gently with two or three fingers the pulse at the carotid artery at one side of the neck. Others take it at their wrists. Again, be sure to count zero as you start, and then 1, 2, 3 etc. You can take your rate for 10 seconds or 15 seconds. I prefer taking my heart rate for 15 seconds and doubling twice to get the rate.

2. If you have not been exercising regularly, see your doctor. Have the doctor examine and approve you for exercise. A discussion of the pro's and con's of various aerobic exercise methods follows in Chapter 15.

3. Select a cardiofitness type exercise you like. It can be any cardio-effective exercise as sufficiently brisk walking, slow jogging, swimming, treadmill, exercise bicycle, etc. You always can change exercise method if needed, or use more than one type of exercise.

    It can be useful to do two or more kinds of exercise such as swimming and walking or treadmill and bicycle. Each builds up somewhat different muscles. The heart does not care what exercise is making it beat faster. If a convenient exercise program does not produce the two hours of time needed, you can finish the needed time with some fast walking once you become reasonably cardiofit.

4. Identify a highest heart rate that you now maintain over time during either your regular physical exercise or walking. If you do not exercise now, take your heart rate after at least three minutes of walking at the most brisk pace you use for walking a significant distance. This will be a starting heart rate level for your exercise.

5. Select the time and frequency of exercise sessions. Examples meeting the desirable two hour time per week could be 6 sessions of 20 minutes, 4 sessions of 30 minutes, 3 sessions of 40 minutes, etc. But at the start you can exercise for lesser times per week if you are not now cardiofit. Exercise time is the time spent exercising at an adequate measured exercise heart rate. This time does not include times for warm-up, cool-down or dressing.

    If you already are exercising in a heart-rate-monitored program such as aerobic dancing or Curves or the equivalent, and develop heart rates of above 110 beats per minute or 18 to 20 per 10 seconds, you may already be doing a CARDIO 120 program. You can skip the step 6 and step 7 that follow. If you are doing such a program but at a lower exercise heart rate than 110 to 120, consider moving up carefully to the needed exercise heart rate. You also will may have to use somewhat more time of exercise than is normally included in versions of these exercise programs to meet the desirable two hours per week of actual cardio exercise.

    People that have confirmed low resting heart rates of 80 or higher may have to exercise to heart rates up to the 130 range to obtain sufficient heart rate elevation. Hopefully, after such exercise is done for several months these high resting rates may decline somewhat.

6. If you are not now exercising, start a first exercise session. Your objective is to exercise at the heart rate you determined from Step 4 above. A heart rate at a given exercise level usually will move up gradually to a plateau rate during a time of 2-3 minutes at a given intensity. Thus you should check its rate after two to three minutes time and occasionally thereafter. Adjust your exercise effort to maintain this desired heart rate.

You can start your first exercise sessions by walking briskly or at the rate found in Step 4 above. You always can change over to another exercise later. If you become tired, stop and rest. Do not push yourself hard when exercising for health. Your exercise always should feel comfortable.

7.   After two weeks at the starting heart rate, increase your exercise heart rate by about 5 beats per minute, if it is less than 120 beats per minute, or 20 in ten seconds. This can be an increase of one in the ten second rate as say from 15 to 16. Continue to increase your heart rate this same amount after each two weeks until you reach the target exercise heart rate of 120 beats per minute or 20 in 10 seconds. This now is your desired exercise program to be continued indefinitely. If you have trouble getting your heart rate up, spend more time at each exercise heart rate level.

8.   When a session time is done, slow down gradually for a while, and walk around a bit after you are finished. Most monitored programs include more than sufficient warm-up and cool-down time.

The time for CARDIO 120 is much less than the frequently recommended time of 3 to 3½ hours for walking. But this two hours per week can still be considerable for many people and is longer than often has been suggested for cardio exercise. The two hours that are useful can be developed in sessions of any length as from 10-12 minutes to a full hour. It might be best to schedule three 40 minutes sessions on alternate days such as Monday, Wednesday and Friday because some research suggests a day of rest between exercise days can be helpful.

But six 20 minute sessions on six days also can be a convenient program with exercise done each morning before breakfast or at some other fixed time. As will follow, there is nothing magic about that two hours. This is just the maximum time that is useful for improving health. You can exercise for a somewhat lesser time and still get useful health benefit. Table 5-1 following shows the benefits from exercising just one hour each week at various exercise heart rates. Appendix 1 shows the cardiofitness improvements obtainable from doing less than the two hours per week maximum.

A full exercise program should include some resistance exercise. If you do 40 minutes per week of resistance exercise you should try to accomplish this with some useful elevation in your exercise heart rate. If you can accomplish this, you can reduce the time at aerobic exercise to say 1½ hours per week. More on this follows later.

Warm-up and Cool-down

CARDIO 120 is a moderate intensity program of exercise at the level of a very brisk or fast walk. Most advice such as five to ten minutes each for warm-up and cool-down probably was intended for much more intensive exercise than this. I don't think many people go through a fancy five or ten minute warm-up and another five or ten minute cool-down and stretching program both before and after a daily very brisk walk home from the station after a commute. Some of the exercise experts tell us we always must do this type of a warm-up after any exercise.

You should do some stretching and warm-up before and after any exercise program. Anyone that has had heart disease or other related medical problem should be guided on this by advice from a doctor. This book is based on what research really tells us about the health value of exercise, and research tells us close to nothing about the health benefits of warm-up or cool-down from moderate exercise and zero about how much time is needed for this. I always work up gradually and slow down gradually for a while at the start and end of fast walking or moderate swimming. I always do some calf stretches and knee bends after fast walking. More on this is in Chapter 15.

Start Using a Trainer or Attending a Class

If you never have exercised regularly, it is best to start a new program using either a group exercise program or a professional trainer. This gives you a time and date for your exercise that helps your compliance. A program such as Aerobic Dancing or Curves can get you accustomed to taking heart rates, and these programs can provide direct CARDIO 120 programs for you if you keep your heart rates at 110-120 per minute or 18 to 20 per 10 seconds. It may require some practice before you can do this comfortably.

A professional trainer is more expensive but can help you in many ways that are not possible from reading a book. Most trainers are experienced in and emphasize resistance training that inherently requires the most teaching. It is excellent to learn about and do this too, but keep in mind as I will show later that the first 1½ to 2 hours per week of aerobic training of the cardiovascular system is of primary importance to health. Your exercise program for health should first emphasize aerobic exercise.

Many combination exercise programs have used only one hour per week of cardio, which is useful but is not sufficient for best health protection. More on benefits of exercising just one hour each week follows.

A purpose of CARDIO 120 is to identify a specific program that will be as simple as possible for people to use and that will help nearly everyone. Past recommendations to walk all or most days of the week required 3 to 3½ hours or more per week. Recognizing how people now usually walk, this recommendation probably will develop a probable average improvement in cardiofitness of about 6-7 CFR. Cardio 120 that produces the first or 10% goal for cardiofitness improvement should more than double this health benefit for a lesser two hours per week. If cardio feedback develops properly, the benefit from Cardio 120 could triple the health benefits obtained from those recommendations to walk.

Managed Cardio

If you have not been exercising regularly and do not intend to exercise in a supervised program, you probably should start exercise first by walking more. Then move to a CARDIO 120 program that can include brisk or fast walking or a variety of other exercises. A Managed Cardio program is another option for those that already have been doing regular exercise.

The first five steps in developing a CARDIO 120 program apply to developing a Managed Cardio program. These involve knowing your Low Resting Heart Rate, how to measure your Exercise Heart Rate, being approved for exercise by your doctor, and selecting your kinds and types of exercise. Follow Steps 1 through 5 for CARDIO 120 and continue following with Step 6.

6.   Get your probable maximum heart rate and maximum desirable exercise heart rate. Write down and remember these numbers. The common 220 minus age formula develops heart rates that are too low for older people. Other more accurate formulas have been developed. The table in Appendix 4 provides these rates from what may be the most accurate available formula. Heart rates at 90% of maximum are 160, 155, 149, 142 and 136 for ages 40, 50, 60, 70, and 80 respectively. It is recommended that you do not attempt to exercise higher than these rates. This step was not needed for CARDIO 120 because a 120 heart rate usually is usable for those of all ages

7.   Identify the highest usual heart rate that you maintain regularly dur-

ing your exercise. If you do not know this, please get this heart rate the next time you exercise. You must know your usual exercise heart rate and be able to monitor this to develop a Managed Cardio program.

8. Select a Master Table appropriate for your low resting heart rate in Appendix 1. Read off the value of CFR shown at the value of your usual exercise heart rate. Example: Your low resting heart rate is 60. Your usual exercise heart rate is 115 average or 19 in ten seconds. Read the value of 18 CFR at a 115 exercise rate from the Appendix 1 Table for a 60 low resting heart rate. If you exercised or intend to exercise for forty weeks or more for 2 hours or more per week, this is a likely contribution of your exercise to your cardiofitness.

    If you have usually exercised less than 2 hours a week, multiply this CFR by the factor for exercise duration that appears following the table. You now have an estimate of the cardiofitness in CFR that your present exercise should be producing over a year term.

9. If you are exercising aerobically more than two hours per week and are exercising for health or weight, you should reduce your aerobic exercise to two hours and consider transferring the exercise time above two hours to resistance exercise. But there is no problem with exercising more than two hours if you wish. There will be some, if quite small, further health benefit and a small contribution to reduction in weight.

10. The CFR value from Step 8 above provides an estimate of your present gain in cardiofitness. This gives you a basis for managing your exercise program. You should aim for at least a 20 CFR value of gain from exercise to attain a good cardio health objective. If your gain is this 20 CFR or more, fine. You probably are developing good benefits.

    If your gain is less than 20 CFR, you should plan to reach this objective if possible. There are three options: First is to increase your time of exercise if you are now exercising less than two hours per week. Second is to increase your exercise heart rate. And third, if you prefer to not increase your heart rate, keep exercising faithfully at your present exercise heart rate to eventually obtain the cardio feed back that also might reduce your low resting heart rate and improve your CFR.

    The Master Table will suggest directly the exercise heart rate you need to use to obtain the needed 20 CFR improvement once you exercise at the two hour per week optimum. If you wish to move to this higher heart rate, you should consider moving the rate up slowly by steps of 5 beats per minute or at one beat per 10 or 15 seconds each month. You cannot go higher than the above guides for maximum heart rate.

11. Your objectives with Managed Cardio are wide open. The first improvements of 10% to 20% in cardiofitness will produce the largest reductions in risk of disease. But further increases in cardiofitness to 30 and even 40 CFR will reduce risks of disease further and continue to improve longevity. I show later that attaining such high levels of cardiofitness also can be a major aid in exercising for weight reduction.

I also will show later some methods for actually measuring your CFR. Many people will have a genetic disadvantage of 10 or even 20 in CFR from an average population value. If you have such a genetic disadvantage, even when doing some useful exercise you may wish to aim for a 30 to 40 improvement in CFR to eliminate the serious potential risk of this genetic factor. A key to this is to keep continually exercising at a measured heart rate to develop the cardio feedback that might move your low resting heart rate down and your cardiofitness up to these high levels.

Cardio of One Hour Per Week

A common recommendation today by many exercise experts is to do 20 minutes of so-called cardio three times each week. With a monitoring of heart rate, this becomes a Managed Cardio program. One hour each week of good cardio exercise can be an excellent program if exercise heart rate can be maintained comfortably at about 50 to 60 beats per minute above low resting heart rate. But one hour per week is only half of the optimal cardio time. I show in Table 5-1 the average improvement in CFR that will be estimated from the appended Master Tables for just one hour of exercise.

For the usual person starting exercise, who has a low resting heart rate of about 70 beats per minute, a cardio exercise heart rate of 130 for the one hour per week should produce the first or 10% improvement in cardiofitness. The exercise heart rate of 160 rate needed for a 20% would not be feasible for persons above age 40. See Appendix Table A5-1 for maximum feasible heart rates. Persons with this low starting CFR probably should not use an exercise heart rate above 130.

Table 5-1

IMPROVEMENT in CFR for ONE HOUR PER WEEK of CARDIO EXERCISE			
Basis: Starting CFR 90-100 One Year of Exercise			
Low Resting Heart Rate	50	60	70	80
Exercise Heart Rate	Improvements in CFR Represent Percent Increases in Cardiofitness		
100	11	6	3	1
110	14	9	5	3
120	18	10	7	5
130	23	12	10	7
140	27	19	13	9
150	33	23	17	11
160	38	27	20	14

But as cardiofitness improves and low resting heart rate moves down, many individuals can obtain a good 20% or better improvement in cardiofitness from one hour per week of exercise at feasible exercise heart rates. Those with a low resting rate of only 50 can obtain a good 20% improvement with one hour of cardio exercise using a heart rate of only about 125. Those with a 60 resting heart rate can obtain this good improvement at an exercise heart rate a bit above 140.

Those that cannot reach a desired goal with the one hour week have the option of increasing their time of exercise up to the two hour per week maximum. This could increase the above one-hour gains in cardiofitness by up to about 75%. See the Master Tables to estimate a likely improvement in cardiofitness for any combination of exercise heart rate and its duration. Continued exercise after a year at a monitored heart rate should reduce your low resting heart rate and improve significantly the gain in CFR you can achieve from working at a given exercise heart rate.

A presumed increase in risk of heart attack may accompany higher exercise heart rates. I found no useful research on this, but that does not deny the possibility. Some exercises such as running produce substantially more injuries than do more moderate exercise. Swimming, walking on an inclined treadmill and bicycle may have lesser risks than running when exercising at high heart rates. More on this follows later.

This ends the steps for doing Managed Cardio.

Obtaining a Cardiofitness Genetic Factor

Some individuals have different genetics in regard to cardiofitness and have a lower than usual cardiofitness for age. Others become reasonably cardiofit from rather little exercise. The new Master Table method provides a first method for estimating one's Genetic Factor for cardiofitness.

The approach is first to estimate the cardiofitness from usual exercise and add this to the usual cardiofitness of 90 CFR for inactive persons. This will provide an estimate of an average person's cardiofitness from exercise and lifestyle. This value is then compared with a measured value of cardiofitness in CFR developed as in Part 2 and Appendix 2. The ratio as percentage of actually measured CFR to the estimated CFR provides a measure of genetic susceptibility. The specifics for doing this are cited further in Appendix 1

A person that has a low cardiofitness genetic factor has an added incentive to reduce this risk through more exercise. The identification of what can be a very high health risk from cardiofitness suggests that particular care is needed in observing other health factors such as diet.

Interval Exercise

There has been much hype recently about interval exercise. This means exercise at alternating higher and lower exercise heart rates as opposed to exercising at one similar heart rate. A sizeable portion of all exercise has been done at differing intensities. Circuit training at different exercise stations, which I did in the 1970's, does this. Aerobic dancing involves rests between exercises. For years I exercised alternately walking fast with periodic jogging. This is interval exercise.

There must be a million ways to do interval exercise. But a recent fad has been doing interval exercise on a treadmill. One of these ways was used in a recent research study.[81] The participants exercised alternately for 1 minute at a high level followed by one minute at a much lower level. Another group used 2 minutes sessions at each exercise rate. The result of this interval exercise was compared with that of a group doing exercise at a steady intermediate rate. The interval groups won.

The Heart Theory explains why this should happen. Cardiofitness develops from the highest intensity maintained for time. If the interval training were carried out long enough, the highest exercise level maintained for 2 hours a week will produce the resulting cardiofitness. Recall what happened in the research shown in Figure 3-1 in Chapter 3 and in other confirming studies of exercise intensity.

If the higher level of interval exercise is one that can be comfortably maintained, there would be no purpose in exercising at a lower rate. This would only reduce the cardiofitness level obtained.

But suppose that the high level of an interval exercise is one that cannot be sustained for the full time of exercise. Interval exercise at these intensities could enable a person to reach a higher cardiofitness than that possible from a highest lower level that could be sustained. As per the Heart Theory this interval exercise then should produce a slightly higher cardiofitness. The Heart Theory method may have a capability for computing the likely results from any kind and combination of interval exercise.

A problem here is that vigorous interval exercise at levels beyond those that can be maintained may be appropriate for athletes or other fitness mavens seeking to reach very high cardiofitness. But such highly vigorous interval exercise does not seem to be the most appropriate training for average people that are exercising to improve their health.

There is talk about a spurt of aerobic energy creating an anaerobic debt because heart rates will not increase fast enough to supply the needed energy. All fairly vigorous aerobic exercise seems to create an anaerobic debt. This can be viewed by carefully recording resting heart rates that follow aerobic exercise sessions at intervals for an hour or two, and comparing these rates with your usual resting heart rate during a day. See the Figure 4-1 in Chapter 4. If the heart rate following exercise remains higher than your usual resting heart rate, this will identify an energy burn that is not measured during the time of exercise per se.

If we identify some useable and comfortable heart rate as a maximum desired for safety or other reason, it is optimum to exercise steadily at this rate. Interval exercise can only produce a loss in effectiveness. If you find interval exercise more enjoyable, by all means do it. But I suggest you forget about the idea that this is some magic bullet that can measurably reduce your weight more or will further improve your health by very much.

I next describe a very simple method for monitoring your cardiofitness that can tell you when your exercise is sufficient to produce good health goals. It is called Cardiofitness Points.

CHAPTER 6

CARDIOFITNESS POINTS CAN MAKE LIFE BETTER

Back in 1968 Kenneth Cooper published his classic Aerobic Point method for developing the exercise needed for cardiofitness. Many thousands of mostly younger men and women must have tried to get their needed 30 Aerobic Points. Cooper showed the importance of aerobic or conditioning type exercise and why it was so much better than isometric, isotonic, resistance or other anaerobic exercise. The centerfold of his book identified Aerobic Point values for doing various vigorous exercises such as running or swimming in stated amounts of time. You needed 30 Aerobic Points to reach his demanding goal for cardiofitness.

The method could be complicated and not easy to use. But it seems well-tested and probably was accurate. His 30 Aerobic Points, if maintained, probably would have improved cardiofitness by at least 25% or 25 CFR and produced a major health benefit. Although a vast amount of research has been done since, I see no similar useful update of this method in the literature. Aerobic Points seem now to be long forgotten.

I propose here a new and quite different point method called Cardiofitness Points. My method accomplishes the same purpose as did Cooper's Aerobic Points but is far easier to use. It tells how much exercise is needed to develop useful health goals for cardiofitness.

What Are Cardiofitness Points?

Cardiofitness Points (CP) value the benefits of cardio exercise from heart rate monitored exercise. I consider a first or basic example for exercise sessions of 30 minutes each because this is a common duration of monitored exercise sessions. It is popular to obtain exercise heart rates from 10 second measurements in Aerobic Dancing and Curves and some other exercise programs. Thus Cardiofitness Points are designed to use these 10 second heart rates.

Cardiofitness Points are simply the difference between your average ten-second exercise heart rate and your ten-second low resting heart rate multiplied by the number of exercise sessions done each week. This is a direct measure of the additional amount of blood your heart is pumping. Points accumulate only for exercise of a first two hours per week. More on this and some examples follow.

Getting Those Cardiofitness Points

You first should obtain your low resting heart rate measured in 10 seconds. It is best to measure your low resting heart rate in beats per minute as a described in Chapter 4. Then divide the beat per minute value by 6 to obtain the rate in 10 seconds. Or you can take your resting heart rate for periods of just 10 seconds in the morning before breakfast after sitting quietly for a few minutes, and repeat this measurement several times to be sure you obtain an accurate average value.

Most people will have a value for their 10-second low resting heart rate of either 10, 11 or 12. If you do not know your low resting rate now, start by assuming a value of 11. You always can check that value later. Again, always start your heart rate count with a zero.

Let's try Example #1 Suppose your low resting heart rate in ten seconds as described above is 12. You exercise for 30 minutes and your 10 second exercise heart rate averages about 18 during this session. You exercise four sessions of this 30 minute program each week.

You subtract the 12 for the 10-second low resting heart rate from the 18 for your 10 usual second exercise heart rate. This gives you 18 minus 12, or 6 Points for the exercise session. You multiply this 6 points per session times the 4 sessions per week. This gives you a total weekly Points of 24. Because your low resting heart will change only very slowly over many months, you usually will need only to estimate only your exercise heart rate when developing Cardiofitness Points. You should re-check your low resting heart rate every few months.

Table 6-1 following shows you that you need 28 Points to reach over time the first goal of a 10% improvement in cardiofitness from 30-minute exercise sessions. If you increase your usual exercise heart rate from 18 (that was only 108 beats per minute) to 19, (or 114 beats per minute) you would develop 7 Points each session and meet your goal of 28 Points each week in only the same four exercise sessions. In this example and as will follow you cannot benefit by exercising more sessions per week because the four present sessions produce the maximum effective duration for exercise of two hours each week.

Table 6-1

Cardiofitness Points required for Exercise Sessions of Different Length Maximum Exercise Time of 2 Hours per Week			
Exercise in Minutes per Session	Maximum Sessions Per week	Points for First Goal, CFR of +10%	Points for Good Goal, CFR of +20%
15	8	56	80
20	6	42	60
30	4	28	40
40	3	21	30
60	2	14	20

For Example 2, suppose your exercise of 30 minutes each session averages at the 20 per ten-second rate. This is an exercise heart rate of 120 beats per minute. Assume for this example that your low resting rate is 11 in ten-seconds. In this example, 20 minus 11 or 9 Cardiofitness Points earned for the 30-minute session. Now just three 30-minute sessions of this exercise would produce 27 or close to the first goal for cardiofitness improvement. Four sessions of this would give you 36 Points each week. This is nearly sufficient to reach the good goal for cardiofitness that from Table 6-1 requires 40 Points

It usually is more convenient to obtain additional Cardiofitness Points by increasing usual exercise heart rate than by increasing numbers of exercise sessions. But this should be done only if this exercise is comfortable. As you exercise more, your cardiofitness should improve, and this should help you gain Cardiofitness Points by both reducing the resting heart rate value and improving attainable exercise heart rates.

As always, you cannot count exercise that totals more than two hours per week. For 30-minute sessions this means that you can count only up to four sessions each week.

Cardiovascular Points for Different Times of Exercise

You may prefer to exercise at other than 30 minutes per session. Or the program you exercise in does not produce exercise for 30 minutes. You then need to develop different targets needed for your Cardiofitness Points. Table 6-1 shows the number of Points you need for exercise sessions of different times and the maximum number of these sessions that can be counted for Cardiofitness Points

For example, if you exercise only 15 minutes per session, it will take twice as many sessions to reach the same exercise time as those from 30-minute sessions. You thus need twice as many Points to reach the same overall time as those from 30-minutes sessions.

You need to remember only the Cardiofitness Points goal needed for your usual exercise time per session. Keep in mind that those times are for the time that you are actually exercising. You cannot count warm-up and other time spent not exercising during the exercise session.

The Cardiofitness Point method is not a substitute for the more complete Master Table method. But it can guide people to improve their cardiofitness in a very simple way. Please try getting your Points. It can be fun to learn how you need to exercise to reach really productive goals for your cardiofitness and health.

Getting Cardiofitness Points from Other Exercise

The Cardiofitness Point method was designed to help people in monitored exercise programs measure their progress toward good cardiofitness. But you do not have to participate in a monitored program. You can get your Cardiofitness Points on your own. You also can supplement the exercise done in a group exercise program that totals less than the two hour per week maximum with other exercise you do on your own.

If you walk on a treadmill or do any other cardio exercise for certain times each session, you can get your Points easily. Simply stop and count your heart rate for 10 seconds. Subtract your low resting heart rate for 10 seconds from this exercise heart rate in 10 seconds. Then multiply these Points by the number of similar exercise sessions you do each week. You do need to exercise at sessions of near equal duration to use the goals for Cardiofitness Point listed for different times of exercise in Table 6-1. And you should observe the maximum number of exercise sessions that can be counted for each session time of exercise.

Reduction in Body Weight from Cardiofitness Points

Your Points provide an approximate measure of the energy of your exercise. Thus as you develop more Points you will be burning more calories for weight control. Actual calories burned will depend on your body weight and level of cardiofitness. But you can figure that producing twice as many cardiofitness points also will be generating twice as many calories burned. When exercising for weight, there will no two hour limit for the effectiveness of Cardiofitness Points

Health Benefits from Cardiofitness Points

A next chapter details the outstanding health benefits that accompany improvements in cardiofitness. As before, a first goal of 10% improvement in cardiofitness suggests a reduction in risk of heart disease of nearly in half, and a reduction in risk of most types of cancer, dementia, diabetes, and other major diseases by about 35%. The second or good goal of 20% improvement will reduce risk of heart disease by nearly 4 times, and risks of those other diseases by about 2 ½ times. As before, continuing this exercise for life can add 3 ½ years of healthy days for the first goal and 6 to 7 years of healthy days for the good cardiofitness goal.

No one can predict the future, and no exercise or other health program can prevent some major disease from occurring to some people. But better cardiofitness gives us better odds for staying healthy. Much more on this follows in the next chapter.

And the best of all: Better Cardiofitness can make each day of your life better. You should feel better, move better, and simply feel more alive.

Part Two

Cardiofitness is of Major Importance to Our Health and Life

CHAPTER 7

HOW CARDIOFITNESS REDUCES RISK OF MAJOR DISEASES

We can be overwhelmed today by the mass of information we read about what we should do to improve our health. Every factor seems to be accompanied by a percentage number. We get 27% for doing this and 42% for doing that. It is virtually impossible to learn from this maze of percentages what is important and what is trivia.

Cardiofitness is not just another health factor. This is not something like a reduction of 20% in cholesterol or cutting down on diet salt. Or something like blueberries may be good for us or chocolate is not as bad as we used to think. Unless our overall diet is extremely unhealthful and of highest health risk, no other lifestyle action can produce as much health benefit to us as will the maintaining of good cardiofitness.

This section on how cardiofitness reduces risk of major disease is more extensive than disease risk evidence usually included in books on health. There are two reasons for this.

First, there have been no previous similar reviews of how cardiofitness reduces risks of major disease. Nearly all previous publications have been about exercise, and exercise and cardiofitness can be quite different things. Cardiofitness is vastly more important to health than is what is usually called exercise. The analyses that follow here are global because they include analysis of all published research . They are not based on results from a recent study or two, which is the more usual scope of evidence in many books on health. I provide many new findings, published only here and on my website.

Second, the key problem that can keep us from becoming fit is our motivation. Doing exercise may not always be what we want to do. I ask myself, "Why was I so motivated to exercise that I did this nearly every day of my life for more than three decades?"

My answer is easy. My family history of disease with a father that died at age 45 and both grandfathers that died before 62 was alarming. And the study of the 50 papers about exercise and heart disease that I did back in the 1970's convinced me completely about what I needed to do.

I hope what follows here will help convince you of the importance of good cardiofitness, and that this will help you to do the exercise needed to keep yourself cardiofit for life.

Heart and Cardiovascular Disease

You or a family member probably have had coronary heart disease, or you know a friend who has had it. It is the most important killer of men and women today. You also may know someone that has had a stroke. Both of these major diseases are key parts of what is called cardiovascular disease, our major terminator of life.

More than a hundred studies have now been published relating risk of heart and cardiovascular diseases to physical activity. Nearly all of these results support the academic theory that physical activity reduces risk of heart or cardiovascular disease. But none tells us accurately what kind and amount of physical activity is needed to get useful benefits.

The research about our health habits today is a world of statistics and statisticians. The researchers develop ratios of risk for our different habits. We now have published studies that have developed hundreds of these risk ratios. But little scientific analysis of what these results mean has been done.

We are told incessantly by the media that we "need to exercise." Sadly, during the past decade advice from various sources about how we should exercise has become a mountain of inaccuracy and confusion. Exercise can take a lot of our time and energy. We need to know what exercise really reduces risk of disease, and how much we really need to do.

I described in Chapter 1 the very large associations of risk of heart disease with poor cardiofitness. Chapter 2 showed how different walking amounts of pace and duration could reduce risk of this important disease.

The following describes in more depth the striking and probable casual relationship of the risk of heart and cardiovascular disease to Cardiofitness Ratio, or the CFR. This CFR measures the risk of disease far more usefully than does any other measure of our exercise.

I first learned this back in the 1970's when studying the research then available. The different kinds of exercise that produced the largest differences in health risk seemed to be those that would best produce what physiologists then called cardiovascular fitness. A factor for this fitness that I now call the CFR explained the risk of all types of heart disease and death from all causes. As mentioned, I published these relationships in The Pulse Point Plan in 1982. I reproduce those first discovered relationships in Appendix 7. But those early values for the CFR that were so well related to risk of heart disease all were estimated. No study then had been published relating actually measured values of CFR to risk of disease.

The Studies of Cardiofitness and Health

A powerful confirmation of the importance of cardiofitness came later in the 1980's with the results of Lie, Ekelund, Arraiz, Blair and others. These studies showed that groups that had low measured values of cardiofitness had dramatically higher risks of heart disease than did those that had high measured cardiofitness. The relationships they obtained for cardiofitness and risk of heart disease confirmed almost exactly the ones I had published earlier.

This 1980's research, as shown in Table 1-1 of Chapter 1, showed order of magnitude larger risks and benefits for differences in measured cardiofitness than has been obtained from studies of what was called physical activity. I noted that Paffenbarger found a 1.7 times risk of heart disease associated with 2,000 average physical activity calories per day. But Blair found a vastly higher 7.9 times difference in risk from a lesser 1,450 calories of cardiofitness. The words exercise, physical activity and cardiofitness thus can have vastly different meanings.

A problem – and in fairness to the many observers who still do not realize the importance of this research about cardiofitness – is that most of it was presented in research papers according to a statistical dogma that produced results of little use to people. Most of the researchers buried their important findings in what I see as inane and nearly useless statistics. They failed to communicate their important findings to the public.

A usual study of measured cardiofitness first involved selection of thousands of people. Each participant's actual cardiofitness was measured, usually with a difficult and expensive test designed to estimate their VO2 Max. This test usually required each participant to exercise to near exhaustion. Now a logical thing to do was to measure how those at low, middle and higher cardiofitness levels related to risk of disease and death in a following period. This would tell us directly how our health risk related to cardiofitness levels that could be duplicated by people. Right?

No. This is not what the statisticians did. They put those of differing cardiofitness into groups in order of level as 1 through 5. They then showed that group 5 having highest cardiofitness had lower risk than group 1 having the lowest cardiofitness. Most researchers told us little or nothing about the actual cardiofitness of any group. This effectively buried the excitingly important casual relation between cardiofitness and risk of disease. Arguably, this should have been the primary purpose of each study.

These statistical ratios for 'groups' were of minimal help to people beyond confirming that exercise and cardiofitness was "Good." Those in Group 1 stayed healthier than did those in Group 5. But no one could know what group they belonged in or what the results really meant for them.

We can't blame the individual statisticians because this is what they are expected to do by their peers. But there should have been someone long ago to do the elementary analysis I did.

We Can Uncover the Effect of Measured Cardiofitness

The Cooper Institute Group did show directly the effect of cardiofitness. Figure 1-1 from their study data does show clearly the importance of cardiofitness in a way that is useful. And these researchers did provide information in other papers and on request that permitted the results of their research to be converted from the near useless statistical basis of group numbers to actual cardiofitness levels. Although this was not done by the other researchers, I was able find methods for translating the group number results of other studies back to the far more useful actual levels of cardiofitness that were measured.

Arguably, cardiofitness is what the studies really measured, and what I believe should have been shown to us in the other original papers. With this done, we can view directly how risks of disease and death related to specific levels of cardiofitness. I show in a formal scientific paper on my website for those interested the probable cardiofitness levels of each of the groups used in each of the studies as both VO2 Max and CFR, and more about how this analysis was developed.[16]

Figure 7-1 shows directly how risk of cardiovascular diseases are reduced by better cardiofitness. This may be one of the more important relationships yet found in health research on a major health risk factor. This relates the risk of cardiovascular disease to levels of cardiofitness from the 12 different available and most useful research study measurements.

Figure 7-1

Risk Ratios of Cardiovascular Disease and Differences in Actual Cardiofitness in CFR

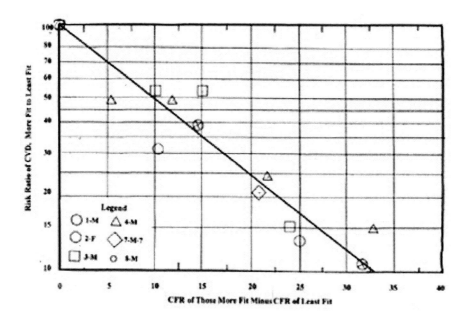

The scale at left shows the %-risk of a heart attack. A value of 100% that represents the risk of each of the sedentary groups of people in these studies is noted at the top left. As we move down the chart, the risk of disease becomes progressively lower. The scale at bottom shows the advantage in CFR of the exercise group minus that of the sedentary group. The line drawn shows that the risk of heart disease becomes progressively lower as the average advantage in CFR of the more cardio-fit group increases. Stated simply, the higher the individual's cardiofitness, the lower the risk of suffering heart or cardiovascular disease.

75

The line drawn touches the bottom of the chart at a risk of heart disease of only 10% or one-tenth at a value of about 33 difference in CFR of cardiofitness. This suggests that if we could improve our CFR level of cardiofitness by 33, or 33%, we should develop a 10 times lower risk of the cardiovascular disease that includes heart disease and stroke.

Each object along the correlation line represents results from studies of from 2,000 to more than 10,000 individuals. Thus this is a global analysis of the large body of available and useful research on cardiofitness. The correlation coefficient is above 0.97. Each increase of 1, or 1%, in cardiofitness reduces risk of heart disease by 6.4%. The same change in risk occurred for both men and women.

If you trace up the correlating line for a 10 difference in CFR, the line shows risk of the exercise group was just 50%, or half of that of the one that did not exercise. At a difference of 20 CFR the risk was down to only 25% of or nearly 4 times lower. As before, I have taken in this book a reduction in risk to 50% as a first goal for a person's desirable improvement in cardiofitness from exercise. A good goal is a 20% improvement in cardiofitness or about a four times lower risk of heart disease.

The above chart suggests that an improvement of 25 CFR that should be achievable by most people would reduce risk of cardiovascular disease to 17% of that of an unfit group. This is a reduction in risk of for heart disease of about 6 times. A really good exercise program can develop up to and beyond the improvement of 33 CFR noted in Figure 7-1 needed for a 10% or ten times lower risk of heart disease. I told in Chapter 4 how I obtained nearly a 50% improvement in cardiofitness from moderate exercise maintained for a period of years.

The results in Figure 7-1 plot as a straight line on what is called semilogarithmic coordinates. This term from engineering suggests a direct casual relationship with each change in CFR having the same percentage effect on risk. It is likely that this type of relationship can be extrapolated with reliability to both much higher and much lower levels than the range shown. This straight line logarithmic relationships greatly increases the importance of this relationship.

The lowest values represented in the plot are for sedentary men and women having a CFR of about 90. But as I will show later, persons that are sedentary with poor genetics may have CFR values ranging down to 70. And athletes with good genetics can gain CFR values 60 to 70 units higher than the zero value in this chart. Thus it is conceivable that the CFR could identify risk levels for coronary disease far larger than the approximately 10-to-1 range measured to date, and ranging up to at least 30-to-one and possibly to 100-to-one.

Although most differences in cardiofitness probably are due to differences in cardio-effective exercise, genetics or family risk can cause some people to have higher innate risks than others. A measurement of cardiofitness identifies both the effects of exercise and any accompanying effect of genetics on risk. I will show later that this cardiofitness is an independent health-risk factor more important than cholesterol, blood pressure, and perhaps even that of heavy smoking.

About Health Risk Ratios:

Health studies sometimes report risks as high ratio divided by low ratio and other times report risks as low ratio divided by high ratio. This book usually uses the high over low ratio that identifies higher risks as 'bad'. Figure 7-1 uses the reverse or low over high ratio. I prefer the high over low basis as identifying risk more realistically. But each doubling of this risk indicates an approximately equal loss in years of life to equal risk of disease. For example, a twice higher risk of heart disease might identify its likelihood at an 8 year earlier time. An increase in risk of four times would suggest that the disease would occur 16 years sooner.

Cardiofitness and Risk of Cancer

Cancer may be our most feared disease. Breast cancer for women, prostate cancer for men or colon or rectal cancer for anyone can strike without little or no warning. Yet at least three-fourths of today's cancer cases do not have to happen. They can be avoided by carefully targeted diet and exercise.

Much research has been done relating the risk of cancer to exercise. Yet the importance of this has been so sparsely published that that few people – and this includes doctors and health experts – realize what this research shows. We see occasional media items about research study results as "Exercise may reduce risk of colon cancer" or "Exercise might reduce risk of breast cancer." The publicity does not tell us how much we need to exercise to obtain some useful reduction in risk. It usually cites only a risk ratio for one type of cancer from some vaguely defined exercise. This kind of information can fail to gain our attention.

A dozen years ago I started as part of my Life Ahead research project to search out, keep track of and organize all of the useful published research results relating physical activity to risk of cancer. As with my earlier compilation of the research relating exercise to heart disease, I was again astounded by how much research had actually been done. My website now tabulates 91 different useful comparisons of exercise and cancer risk from 53 studies. The scientific paper "Exercise, Cardiofitness and Cancer" provides the actual analyses and these individual study data.[46]

Questions not previously answered are: How much benefit can exercise produce in reducing risk of cancer? What kinds of exercise protect best? Is cardio type exercise or just lots of lower intensity exercise such as usual walking best? How does exercise change risk of different types of cancer?

Exercise, Physical Activity and Cancer

A conclusion from all of this sometimes confusing research is that both physical activity of occupation and leisure time provides protection against cancer. Some studies found that exercise early in life provided protection in combination with more recent exercise. For example, those athletic in their youths obtained some residual protection later in life.

The kind and amount of exercise was poorly identified in most of the studies on cancer. We do not have the more concise pace- and duration-related results of walking that we have for heart disease. But it is evident that the correct kind of exercise can substantially reduce our risk of cancer.

Cardiofitness – and Not Just Exercise Calories – Provides the Best Protection from Cancer

The few studies that included an actual measurement of the CFR appeared to identify much larger reductions in risk of cancer than did studies that identified only 'exercise.' For example the Cooper Institute study that is the classic on cardiofitness found a four-fold reduction in risk of all cancer for high cardiofit men and a ten-fold reduction in risk for high cardiofit women. These were far higher levels of protection than those found for lesser quantified amounts of cardio exercise. Arraiz found only a 17% lower cancer risk for differences in participants amounts of what was called exercise, but nearly a 50% lower cancer risk for those that passed a simple step fitness test on the same population.

To answer this question further, I compared the risks of cancer with differences the physical activity calories and cardiofitness values in CFR for each of 89 comparisons of cancer benefit found. Values of cardiofitness were estimated for the studies that did not include actually measured CFR values.

The risk of cancer was related to cardiofitness in CFR at the very high level of 78%. The relation of cancer risk to physical activity calories was a much lower 41%. This shows that cardiofitness produced by exercise explains the risk of getting some type of cancer far better than does physical activity calories of exercise. Yet the Cooper study suggested that my risk of cancer from cardiofitness still may be much too conservative.

This does confirm that the higher intensity exercise that protects best against heart diseases also protects best against cancer. Thus if we design our exercise to protect against heart disease we probably also will obtain best protection against cancer. Most of the values for cardiofitness had to be estimated. The average risks from these estimated values was the same as that from actually measured values. This further verifies the overall conclusions obtained.

The Risk of Different Types of Cancer Are Similarly Reduced by Cardiofitness

Most research studies of cancer are for just one type, as for example colon, breast or prostate. A next question becomes, How do the risks of various types of cancer respond to changes in cardiofitness in CFR? I was surprised to discover that higher cardiofitness reduced the risk of each type of cancer similarly.

Table 7-1 lists at the left the change in risk of different types of cancer per unit change in CFR. It shows at right the number of studies of this type of cancer that were used in obtaining the values. The risks of each type of cancer appeared to be reduced similarly by an improvement in cardiofitness. An average 4% reduction in cancer risk was obtained for each unit increase in cardiofitness in CFR.

Table 7-1

Table 7-1		
Reductions in Risk of Cancer vs. Cardiofitness in CFR		
Cancer Cause	Avg Reduction in Risk per unit increase in CFR	Number of Research Comparisons
Any Cancer	3.7%	11
Colorectal Cancer	3.3%	12
Prostate Cancer	3.9%	8
Breast Cancer	4.5%	31
Endometrial & Ovarian	4.4%	13
All comparisons	4.0%	89

Note that these values for cancer risk by cancer type are each based on the averages of from 8 to 31 different research study comparisons. Risks for lung and pancreatic cancer are not included because of the few comparisons available. But risks for these per increase in CFR also were similar to those in Table 7-1. Cardiofitness reduced the risk of breast cancer most significantly.

It thus seems likely that the exercise that produces cardiofitness also reduces all major causes of cancer similarly. To my knowledge, this is the only comprehensive published comparison of exercise or cardiofitness risks yet developed for different types of cancer.

This reduction in risk of cancer of 4% per CFR is not as high as is the protection of 6.4% per CFR reduction in risk for heart and cardiovascular diseases. But this still is an important protection. For example, an improvement in CFR of 10% that is achievable from fast walking at 4 miles per hour for 2 hours per week will reduce risk of all cancer by nearly 50%. Developing the 20-25% improvement in cardiofitness that is potential from a good cardio exercise program should reduce cancer risk by 2 to 2½ times.

Reducing Cancer Risk May Require Exercise over a Long Time

Good cardiofitness and its protection against heart disease usually can be developed in six months time. This protection can be lost in a similar period of physical inactivity. But protection against cancer may require exercise over much longer time periods.

Some of the research suggests that it might require at least 10 years of exercise to develop a good level of protection for cancer. Protection achieved in earlier years may persist in part into the future. For example, it can take 20 or more years of smoking for cancer to start developing from cigarettes. And it usually takes 10 years for risk to drop back again after smoking is stopped. Exercise for best benefits must be maintained over an entire lifetime. This will be especially true for protecting ourselves from cancer.

Another question is, Does the two-hour exercise time that is most time-effective for heart disease also apply to the exercise for reducing risk of cancer? I could find no answer to this from any of the research on cancer. Useful data comparing the benefit of 2 hours of exercise vs. that for the same intensity at say 4 or more hours of exercise was simply not found.

But risk of cancer is best related to changes in cardiofitness and more than two hours per week of exercise does not improve cardiofitness further. Thus I would not waste time doing aerobic exercise of more than two hours a week for the reduction of cancer risk unless I had a serious weight problem.

The Mechanisms by Which Cardiofitness Protects Against Cancer

A variety of suggested mechanisms have been suggested for the reduction of cancer risk from exercise. But at this writing none of these hypotheses appears to have been verified. The finding that cardiofitness protects best means that high intensity exercise reduces cancer risk more effectively than does low intensity exercise. This suggests that the higher flow of blood in the cardiovascular system from cardio exercise disperses a protective agent more effectively throughout the body.

The new finding that cardio exercise reduces risk of different types of cancer similarly suggests that a common agent distributed more effectively by the higher blood flow of cardio exercise protects all body cells from cancer. Much of the nutrition needed for the body is carried by the blood, and higher intensity exercise pushes blood flow more efficiently throughout our vast circulatory system of arteries, capillaries and veins. This same higher flow of blood maintained for some significant time each week also helps keep coronary and other arteries more open.

What is that mysterious agent in our blood that may be protecting our cells from developing all kinds of cancer? Selenium is one possibility. But our blood includes dozens of nutrients that could protect against cancer. A multiplicity of nutrients could be involved.

Diabetes

Diabetes can be a curse that significantly diminishes the quality of life. It imposes restricted eating habits that reduce the joy of food. Many have to take daily blood samples to test their insulin level. Diabetes substantially increases the chance of heart disease, stroke, and other cardiovascular diseases. Many diabetics suffer nerve diseases such as neuropathy that can cause constant and difficult to cure pain. And diabetes is difficult or impossible to cure. About 7% of the US population has diabetes. A significant number of those that have diabetes are unaware that they have it.

The most important health factor by far that produces diabetes is being overweight. A modest difference in weight of only about 25 pounds increases the risk of diabetes by 14 times at age 50 and an incredible 24 times at age 60. Thus exercise can have a major role in reducing risk of diabetes by helping to reduce weight. More on this will follow.

Exercise helps reduce blood sugar and also helps insulin become more effective in controlling it. The Life Ahead paper on diabetes provides seven risk measurements from four useful studies of the benefits of exercise in reducing the risk of diabetes.[47] The average benefit found was a reduction in risk of about 1/3rd for "regular exercise" that probably improved cardiofitness only modestly.

But the study by Wei of the Cooper Institute indicated that cardiofitness was a more accurate predictor of risk.[48] Measured values of cardiofitness forecast risk better than did self report of exercise. Each increase of 1 unit or 1% in the CFR appeared to reduce risk of diabetes by 5%. This compares with values of 6.4% per CFR for heart disease and 4% per CFR for cancer.

This suggests that an increase of ten in CFR from a quite brisk walking program should reduce diabetes risk by 40%. A 25% increase in CFR from an effective cardio exercise program should reduce risk by more than three times. These values all are for people of a given weight. A much larger benefit from exercise than this probably will develop because weight also is usually reduced by exercise.

The two-hour limit for exercise in improving cardiofitness and reducing risks of most diseases does not apply to those now having diabetes. As cited earlier, the Nurses study found that exercise for more than two hours per week could reduce the risk of heart disease for women with diabetes.[24] This is the only clear exception found in which more than 2 hours per week of exercise was beneficial in reducing risk of a disease. This benefit of more hours of exercise probably is due to the very large effect of exercise in reducing body weight.

Alzheimer's and Dementia

Dementia now strikes nearly a quarter of all older adults. It may be our most rapidly growing national health problem as our population becomes older. This disease diminishes the quality of life of both the sufferer and one or more caregivers. A single case of dementia can involve a loss of quality of life for at least two people for up to 15 or 20 years.

The Life Ahead paper on dementia lists the results of 15 comparisons from 8 useful studies that relate exercise to the risk of suffering this disease.[49] These studies were carried out on older people and involved rather modest amounts of vigorous exercise. Despite this, the average group that exercised more in 15 different test comparisons obtained a 43% average reduction in risk of suffering future dementia.

One study showed that cognitive decline was statistically related to level of cardiofitness. A pattern of the results from all studies suggested that more vigorous activity was most protective. Men who could walk at a higher speed obtained more protection. The kind and amount of exercise in these studies of dementia probably would produce CFR improvements in the order of 5 to 10%. On this basis, an improvement of one CFR or 1% would reduce risk of dementia and Alzheimer's by about 5%. This is a similar to the benefit of cardiofitness in reducing the risk of diabetes.

Exercise that reduces the risk of any disease may only delay its onset to an older age. Most dementia occurs toward the end of life. Thus a reduced risk and deferral to an older age from a proper exercise program can mean that the disease will never happen at all.

Respiratory Disease. or COPD

Respiratory diseases, now called chronic obstructive pulmonary disease (COPD), are the fourth largest cause of death in the US. They rival stroke as a cause of major disabling disease, hospitalization and premature death.[50] COPD includes chronic bronchitis, emphysema, asthma, and some other diseases of the respiratory system. Most of these diseases when present to the extent that hospitalization is needed, may be irreversible.

Individuals often are enrolled in an exercise program designed to improve their lung function after COPD is diagnosed. Research has shown that carefully programmed exercise will usefully improve cardiofitness as measured by a distance walked in 6 or 12 minutes or by other fitness tests. Such programs of cardiofitness improvement done for only a few weeks can improve the condition of some COPD sufferers for two years.

COPD is diagnosed by a measure called FEV1/FVC. A study by Cheng from the Cooper Institute showed a clear relationship between the COPD levels of older people and their measured cardiofitness, with high values of FEV1/FVC being better. Men and women having these higher FEV/FVC were significantly less likely to suffer COPD. This suggests that improved cardiofitness is a likely protector of COPD.

Macular Degeneration

Age Related Macular degeneration (AMD) is an incurable eye disease that it is the leading cause of blindness for those aged 60 and older in the US. It afflicts more than 10 million older Americans and causes more blindness than do cataracts and glaucoma combined. Those with a diagnosis of macular degeneration can no longer drive a car. They can lose their ability to read except with the aid of magnification. Near complete blindness may result later.

I found only two studies of exercise and risk of macular degeneration.[51] But these indicated that cardiofitness was a probable important protector. The first study by Klein, from the important Beaver Dam project, found a risk of 0.27 or nearly a 4-fold reduction in risk of macular degeneration from those that "worked up a sweat five times each week."[52] This definition of exercise suggests good cardio exercise that would produce a likely 15-20% higher CFR.

The second study found a 25% reduction in risk for a general question about more exercise that would identify little more than a 5% - 8% higher cardiofitness. This limited information again suggests a possible benefit of at least 5% in risk for each change of 1 in CFR that is similar to the benefits of cardiofitness in reducing risks of other diseases.

Osteoporosis

Osteoporosis is a disease of declining bone density that can result in fractures of the hip, vertebrae or other bones. Hip fractures can be repaired today, but 20% of those that suffer them die within a year. Fractures of the back vertebrae can result in serious disability. It has long been known that lack of exercise can cause osteoporosis.

Results of 7 good studies of exercise and risk of osteoporosis are listed in a Life Ahead paper. All studies found useful reductions in risk from exercise.[53] The large study of the Nurses showed that walking pace was the primary factor that reduced risk, with walking duration of lesser importance. This identifies a likely effect of cardiofitness. A very brisk walking pace reduced risk ratio for hip fracture to 0.39 for a benefit of 2.6 times.

Although most vigorous cardio-type exercise produced the best benefits, these studies were mostly for younger people that had adequate bone density. As people become older their bone density often declines to levels that are at high risk for hip, vertebrae or other fractures. A prominent factor in such fractures is falls, and one in three people over age 65 appears to suffer one or more falls each year.

Research has demonstrated that those that exercise regularly are less likely to fall. But as people grow older more caution is needed to avoid falls. Thus the most appropriate exercise to reduce risk of osteoporosis for those older may be carefully managed walking. Walking produces most health benefits from its effect in improving cardiofitness.

Arthritis

Another curse of older age is arthritis. It can also happen less frequently to those who are younger. Arthritis involves the reduction or destruction of cartilage that keeps bones from rubbing together. Deficient cartilage often causes pain at the knee, hip, back or hand that can become severe. Arthritis can cause near continual pain and often is incurable. Treatment usually involves medications that reduce but do not eliminate its pain.

Exercise can be either harmful and helpful. Eight studies of exercise and arthritis explain how this can happen.[54] Those subject to serious stress and physical injury could develop arthritis many years later at the location of the injury. Men in heavy physical occupations during earlier years had a much higher risk of getting arthritis later in life.

Yet three of the studies found that those that did more usual exercise reduced risks of getting arthritis. A study of 1300 athletes in Finland found that endurance and track and field athletes had a third to a half of the arthritis suffered later by the average population. Only those involved in contact sports suffered higher risks. Another Finnish study found that those doing running or much walking suffered only a fifth the average number of knee surgeries. And a US study of 2100 people found that the quarter doing the most exercise over a 20 year period suffered one-third less arthritis. The answer appears clear from this research. Regular exercise – and this probably includes exercise of any set of body muscles – should substantially reduce risk of arthritis at these locations. This includes the type of exercise that is most useful for reducing risk of the major cardiovascular diseases and cancer. But falls and injuries from this exercise need to be avoided. Thus reducing risk of arthritis could be obtained best from very brisk walking or swimming.

Will that pounding from running eventually harm our knees, hips or back? Arthritis Research & Therapy in September 2005 showed from a 14-year study of musculoskeletal pain that runners had a far lower incidence of pain than did an average control group. Women runners had a 12% increase in pain vs. 71% increase for controls. Male runners had an 18% increase vs. a 41% incidence for controls.

The foregoing includes most of our very major lifetime health problems. Their risk can be substantially reduced by the exercise that produces cardiofitness. Research has suggested many other ways exercise can help us improve our life, and a few of these will be cited later.

The Risks of Death From All Causes

Reducing risk of heart disease and cancer and other individual diseases can be important. But the ultimate aim of good health is to decrease our risk of that 'ultimate event' that can reduce our healthy life span. Some studies of cardiofitness and risk showed not only risks of cardiovascular diseases but risks of death from all causes.

Figure 7-2 shows from the available research that cardiofitness in CFR reduces the risk of death from all causes. The sedentary groups are represented by that circle at 100% on the left-hand scale. The line drawn shows how risk becomes progressively lower as the CFR of the exercise groups increased. Cardiofitness reduces the risk of death from all causes by 4.6 % for each % increase in our CFR.[16] This relation has a high significance and a correlation coefficient of a very high 96%. This is not a usual plot of research data vs. results. Each point in this chart represents results of an entire research study that in turn included results on several thousand individuals.

This value of a 4.6% reduction in risk for each percentage improvement in cardiofitness is smaller than the 6.4% per percentage improvement in risk per percent increase in CFR found for heart disease, but similar to the reduction on risk obtained for cancer. This still identifies a very large and important improvement in health. An improvement of 10 in CFR for a first goal should reduce risk of death to 60% of average and an improvement of 20 in CFR for the good goal should reduce risk of a death from all causes to 37% of usual, or by nearly three times.

This research supports the finding that an increase of about one-third of a year of added life develops from each improvement of one in the CFR of cardiofitness. Obtaining a 20% improvement in CFR, which is possible from good maintained cardio exercise, would give a middle-aged man or woman about 6-7 more years of healthy days of life ahead. These are not just days added on to the end of a life. They include those many days that the above major diseases were not present and likely diminishing the quality of life.

How Does Cardiofitness Protect Against Death From All Causes?

There has been vast speculation about how exercise produces health benefits. We now have sufficient research that defines quantitatively how some other factors can contribute to cardiofitness. This research can replace some of this speculation with more probable quantified casual factors.

Figure 7-2

Risk Ratios of Death from All Causes and Differences in Actual Cardiofitness in CFR

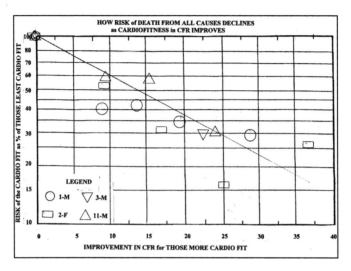

Cholesterol

Improvements in cardiofitness from exercise usually reduce total and LDL cholesterol levels and increase desirable HDL cholesterol levels. It has been widely speculated that cholesterol might explain the effect of exercise on heart disease.

This is not true. These risk factors explain only a very small part of the major benefit that is accomplished by cardiofitness. We now have defined risks of heart disease and death from measured values of cardiofitness at high significance as in Figures 7-1 and 7-2. In order to identify likely causes it is a requirement that each be quantified to explain some part of or all of these overall risk benefits.

Five meta-analyses of exercise and cholesterol showed that exercise reduced total and LDL cholesterol an average 4.2 mg/dl and increased HDL an average of 2.0 mg/dl. But these analyses did not show how cholesterol was changed by differing amounts or kinds of exercise.

Twenty-seven study results from ten studies in the database on exercise and cardiofitness did relate amounts of changes in cholesterol to cardiofitness These showed that both exercise intensity and duration reduced total and LDL cholesterol, with intensity being of most importance.

Table 7-2 shows a quantitative analysis of these results. The values are consistent with results of the meta-analyses but replace their average values of improvement of about 4.2 mg/dl with quantified effects of exercise heart rate elevation above resting heart rate and exercise duration. There was no two-hour limit for the effect of cholesterol as there was for exercise and cardiofitness. From the Master Tables, a 50 beat per minute elevation in heart rate for two hours per week should produce a 13% improvement in CFR, and a reduction in heart disease of 55%.

Each improvement of 1 ml/dl in total or LDL cholesterol reduces risk of heart disease by about 1%. Table 7-2 suggests that at the same heart rate elevation of 50 beats per minute, the reduction in risk from cholesterol would be 3.8%. This 3.8% represents only 7% of the corresponding 55% benefit of cardiofitness in reducing risk of heart disease.

Adding in a benefit for HDL brings the overall change in risk produced by cholesterol to only 10% of the benefit of cardiofitness on heart disease. Some studies have suggested that exercise also reduces triglycerides. Triglycerides at usual levels below 100 to 150 mg/dl vary inversely with HD. Only very high levels of this factor produce added actual risk of disease beyond that associated with HDL.

But cholesterol affects principally only the risk of heart disease. Cardiofitness affects risks not only of heart disease but of most cancer and other causes discussed above in this chapter. These other diseases in total are more important to risk of premature death than is heart disease per se. Overall, differences in cholesterol thus explain less than 5% of the overall health benefits from cardiofitness. The contribution of reducing risk of cholesterol from exercise of more than two hours per week would be too small to be measurable using presently available methods.

Blood Pressure

Blood pressure was reduced slightly by exercise in many different studies. Based on 7 of these studies, each increase of 1 in CFR reduces systolic/diastolic blood pressure by 0.24/0.14 mm. Thus an improvement of 20 in CFR reduces blood pressure an average of about 5/3 mm. This should reduce an average person's cardiovascular risk by about 10%. From Figure 7-1 an increase of 20 in CFR would reduce risk of cardiovascular disease by 75%. Blood pressure could thus explain 13% of this total.

This reduction in blood pressure is a direct and expected casual result of improving cardiofitness. The increased blood flow that produces car-

Table 7-2

Effect of Exercise Intensity and Duration on Changes in Serum Cholesterol						
Heart Rate Elevation beats/minute	Total Cholesterol mg/dl			HDL Cholesterol mg/dl		
	1 Hour/ week	2 hours/ week	4 hours/ week	1 Hour/ week	2 hours/ week	4 hours/ week
30	-0.7	-1.3	-1.7	0.2	0.4	0.7
40	-1.2	-2.4	-3.1	0.3	0.6	1.2
50	-1.9	-3.8	-4.9	0.5	1.0	1.9
60	-2.7	-5.4	-7.1	0.7	1.4	2.7
70	-3.7	-7.4	-9.6	0.9	1.9	3.8
80	-4.9	-9.1	-12.5	1.2	2.5	4

diofitness should open up pathways in the cardiovascular system. As for cholesterol, blood pressure is related mostly to cardiovascular disease. Thus this factor can explain no more that 6% of the overall benefits of cardiofitness.

A question about blood pressure: Blood pressure increases the load on the heart and cardiovascular system. Shouldn't this improve cardiofitness? A probable answer here is that it is the flow of blood induced by exercise that circulates blood most widely throughout the cardiovascular system that enlarges arteries and produces the health benefits of cardiofitness. Blood pressure places an extra load on the heart, but has little if any effect of the actual flow of blood in the system. Further, elevated blood pressure per se has a significant negative effects on both risks of cardiovascular disease and of death from all causes.

C-Reactive Protein or CRP

CRP identifies inflammation that now is a confirmed risk factor. A valuation from the Cooper Institute showed that the most cardio-fit group averaged 0.70 mg/l vs. the least fit group at 1.64 mg/l. This computes to an expected difference in coronary risk of 1.4 times. The actual difference in cardiofitness of these same groups was about 7 times. Thus CRP could explain a part of the effect of cardiofitness but probably no more than a sixth of the total effect on heart disease.

But as for cholesterol, CRP is verified mostly as a risk for heart disease. Recognizing the effect of cardiofitness on a broad range of other diseases shows that it is unlikely that this factor could explain more than 8% of what is explained by cardiofitness.[44]

Another study showed that different types of exercise may have differing effects on CRP. A control group measured 0.5 mg/l. Swimmers obtained 0.1 mg/l, middle runners obtained about 0.3, and racing cyclists and soccer players obtained 0.6. Lower values are associated with lower risk. An inference here is that exercises that disturb the body may produce some increase in risk that could reduce its benefits from cardiofitness.[45]

Keeping Arteries Open

A total of these above known factors might explain 25% of the effect of cardiofitness on heart disease and possibly 15% of an overall health risk associated with cardiofitness. Some other inadequately quantified factors associated with exercise have been speculated as possible causes of its benefits. But by far the most probable casual effect of cardiofitness in reducing risk of coronary heart disease is that the pulsing of increased flow of blood at the elevated heart rates produced by exercise pushes coronary and other arteries more open and circulates blood more thoroughly to body cells.

Figure 7-3

Sections of the main left coronary arteries of monkeys that were fed an atherosclerosis-producing diet for two years

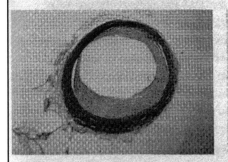 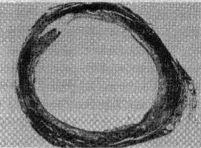

| This animal was kept sedentary. Artery remained small, and hard atherosclerosis closed off 52 percent of the free space available for blood flow needed to fuel the heart muscle. | This animal was exercised. With the comparable artery enlarged to more than twice the size of the artery in the animal that was kept sedentary, a far larger potential blood flow to the heart was provided. |

The remarkable pictures shown here are of the cross sections of the coronary arteries of monkeys. Those having arteries similar to those in the example at left were not exercised, and those having arteries as shown at the right were exercised on a treadmill for one hour, three times each week.[40]

The cross section of the artery of the non-exercising monkey was 50% blocked; the artery at right was enlarged and had far more open cross-sectional area for flow of blood that could prevent a blockage. Most non-exercised monkeys died of coronary disease, but exercised monkeys remained healthy.

This research provided a striking illustration of the power of blood flow from exercise to modify not only the physical structure of the coronary arteries but the likely physical structure of the entire cardiovascular system. This increase in blood flow probably is the defining factor that improves both cardiofitness and the overall capability of the cardiovascular system.

Please study these two photos carefully. The atherosclerosis shown by the grey sections in the left photo was clearly pushed back in the right photo by the higher volume of flowing blood. You can visualize how much more likely the artery at left could be blocked by a blood clot.

I view the results from this study as one of the more important health research findings of the entire 20th century. The example shows clearly how the higher intensity of occasional cardio-effective exercise can keep arteries more open. I showed these results in my previous book, The Pulse Point Plan.

There is little question that this same thing happens to humans. Arteries of men who exercised more were found by a study of Mitrani to be 15% more open.[41] African Masai studied by George Mann that had CFR measured values of 150 had coronary arteries that were 50% larger than usual.[42] A marathoner Clarence DeMar had coronary arteries three times usual size.[43]

An engineering analysis suggests that risk of a blockage would be reduced at least tenfold for a coronary artery enlargement of the magnitude shown in Figure 7-3. This is the only known mechanism that can now explain the very large reductions in risk that accompany improvements in cardiofitness. Because this mechanism involves body muscle, it also explains how coronary risk from a change in cardiofitness can improve in a period of months in response to exercise, and decrease similarly after exercise is stopped.

Viewed overall, it seems likely that about 85% of the health benefits of cardiofitness are due directly to the beneficial effect of higher periodic levels of blood flow on the effectiveness of the cardiovascular system. These same higher blood flows stress the cardio muscle and produce measurable improvements in cardiofitness. These benefits associated with cardiofitness include keeping arteries more open, and distributing nutrients in blood more widely and effectively throughout the body.

Viewed as statistical factors, the remaining 15% of cardiofitness benefits to death from all causes can be attributed to changes in cholesterol factors, blood pressure and CRP. Yet at the more fundamental or casual level most of these statistical benefits also may be produced by cardiofitness. The higher blood flows of cardiofitness that open up cardiovascular system vessels almost certainly are a direct cause of reduced blood pressure. Table 7-2 showed that cardiofitness improved values of cholesterol best. And better cardiofitness reduces levels of CRP. For the health benefit of physical activity calories per se, this leaves only a selective effect in reducing the body weight of the obese.

CHAPTER 8.

Low Cardiofitness is a Major Health Risk Factor

A health risk factor is a measurement of the body that can identify a higher than usual risk of a disease or death. Today's most recognized major risk factors are cholesterol, cigarette smoking, and blood pressure. These are factors that doctors use as warnings about the risks of heart or other disease that a patient is likely to suffer. I show here that cardiofitness can be a more important health risk factor than any of these above recognized risk factors.

Cardiofitness Can Identify a High Health Risk

Cardiofitness usually is thought of as the higher fitness that derives from exercise. A low cardiofitness is something unwanted that is of little interest. Yet importantly, a low level of cardiofitness may identify risk of heart and other major diseases that today is completely overlooked.

The previous chapter showed that cardiofitness can identify a risk of cardiovascular disease of ten times, of cancer up to nearly four times, and of diabetes, Alzheimer's, macular degeneration, COPD and arthritis up to three times. As will be seen, cardiofitness is a risk factor that deserves to be included in physical exams. I show in some following tables that cardiofitness may be the #1 of major risk factors.

93

About the Life Ahead Program

The comparisons of risk that follow are developed using the sophisticated Life Ahead Computer Program. I believe that this now free program is today's most advanced and accurate technology for computing population and individual health risks. The program develops risks and risk of death from 19 different diseases and other factors such as accidents as developed from the US Vital Statistics from age 1 thru 93, with extensions from NIH to age 100 and from other sources to age 110.

All the best and useful studies found published were used in developing risks for diseases. The life-cycle model re-computes all risks at every age of life via an engineering construct that should be much more accurate than conventional statistical type models. A general description of the model is provided. The Life Ahead website (www.lifeahead.net) includes this and provides nearly 100 mostly informal scientific papers describing the construction of the model and the analyses for each included health risk and disease.[55, 56] The comparisons that follow show the risks of heart disease and average US population healthy days of life that are associated with lifetime levels of very high and very low values of each risk factor.

Cardiofitness and Serum Cholesterol

The bold print numbers in the lowest row of Table 8-1 show how health risks associated with large differences in cardiofitness compare with those associated with large differences in total serum cholesterol. The difference

Table 8-1

Table 8-1	Comparison of Health Risks, Cardiofitness vs. Cholesterol for Average US men of age 50					
	Cardiofitness				Total Serum Cholesterol	
CFR	Risk Heart Disease, in next 10 years, %	+Years of Healthy Days of Life		Cholesterol mg/dl	Risk Heart Disease in next ten years, %	+Years of Healthy Days of Life
80	16.3	21.1		300	19.1	22.1
90	12.4	23.1		250	11.4	24.8
100	7.9	26.4		220	8.5	26.1
110	4.8	29.8		200	6.9	26.8
120	2.8	32.8		150	4.1	28.2
Gain:	5.8 times	11.7 yrs		Gain:	4.7 times	6.1 yrs

in cardiofitness is associated with a difference in risk of heart disease of 5.8 times. The difference in cholesterol suggests a somewhat lesser risk of 4.7 times. Higher cardiofitness can contribute 11.7 more years of healthy days; but large differences in cholesterol are associated with a lesser 6.1 more healthy years.

A number of studies suggest that cholesterol levels of 150 are optimum. Values below 150 may increase risk of death. Cholesterol is associated mainly with risks of cardiovascular diseases. Lower cardiofitness values are associated not only with increased cardiovascular risk but also identify higher risks of cancer, diabetes, dementia and other major life terminators described in the previous chapter, which also contribute importantly to long-range health.

As above, the risk comparisons here are for typical US men of age 50 and assume lifetime duration of each risk factor. A change to the different values starting at age 50 would produce lesser changes in risk and years of healthy life ahead than the values shown, but would show similar conclusions. Similar results are obtained from similar comparisons of women.

The health benefits of cholesterol are derived in part from the premier study of J. D. Neaton from the MRFIT program.[57] This massive study included the deaths from coronary disease of 316,000 men for total cholesterol values from 130 to 340 during a subsequent 12-year period.

Today's high values of total and LDL cholesterol can be reduced substantially with the aid of statin-type drugs. Thus the number of people that still have serum cholesterol values above 300 should be small. A much larger estimated 9% of our population may be graded at CFR values of 80 and lower. The only known way for improving their CFR is doing the right amount of cardio-effective exercise.

Cardiofitness and Smoking

Figure 8-2 shows that a large difference in cardiofitness is associated with a 5.8 times higher risk of heart disease. This compares with a 3.4 times higher risk for a man smoking 40+ cigarettes each day. Better cardiofitness is associated with 11.7 years of more healthy life, a value that is about the same as the advantage of 11.4 years for a non-smoker compared with one that did this very large amount of regular smoking.

Risks of smoking were based mostly on the two largest studies of the American Cancer Society. Each of these included results on nearly a million people. But results for some included diseases were based on other key

Table 8-2

Table 8-2	Comparison of Health Risks, Cardiofitness vs. Smoking for Average US men of age 50						
	Cardiofitness				Cigarettes		
CFR	Risk Heart Disease next ten years, %	+Years of Healthy Days of Life			Cigarettes in Number per Day	Risk Heart Disease in next ten years, %	+Years of Healthy Days of Life
80	16.3	21.1			40+	27.9	15.0
90	12.4	23.1			30	22.2	17.2
100	7.9	26.4			15	16.4	20.0
110	4.8	29.8			5	12.1	17.2
120	2.8	32.8			0	8.0	26.4
Gain:	5.8 times	11.7 yrs			Gain:	3.4 times	11.4 yrs

studies of smoking.[58] Not smoking cigarettes benefits health selectively by eliminating the very high risk of lung cancer that occurs for smokers. Better cardiofitness is associated with a larger differences in heart disease than is associated with smoking.

Cardiofitness and Blood Pressure

A large difference in cardiofitness can identify a larger difference in risk than will a large difference in blood pressure.[59] Table 8-3 compares risks associated with cardiofitness with those associated with elevated blood pressure. Note again the bottom line in the table. Differences in cardiofitness

Table 8-3

Table 8-3	Comparison of Health Risks, Cardiofitness vs. Blood Pressure for Average US men of age 50						
	Cardiofitness				Blood Pressure		
CFR	Risk Heart Disease next ten years, %	Years of Healthy Days of Life			Systolic/ Diastolic Pressure	Risk Heart Disease in next ten years, %	Years of Healthy Days of Life
80	16.3	21.1			170/110	21.4	21.0
90	12.4	23.1			150/100	14.1	23.7
100	7.9	26.4			135/85	8.9	25.9
110	4.8	29.8			125/75	6.6	27.0
120	2.8	32.8					
Gain:	5.8 times	11.7 yrs			Gain:	3.2 times	6.0 yrs

can identify higher differences in risk of both heart disease and years of healthy life than do very large differences in blood pressure.

These comparisons each confirm that the presently accepted health risk of cholesterol, cigarettes and blood pressure are very real and large. I have no intention of denigrating these high risks that either individually or in combination can mean much to person's chances of a healthy life.

But these comparisons of objectively and scientifically developed risks show that cardiofitness deserves to be given far more serious attention by our Health Establishment than the near zero attention it is given today. A cardiofitness measurement identifies the physical condition of the heart and its cardiovascular system that includes the most important organs and muscles in our body. I will show that a relatively simple treadmill test should be able to identify cardiofitness usefully.

I showed in the previous chapter that contributions of cholesterol and blood pressure to the overall health benefits of cardiofitness are small. Cardiofitness thus remains as a largely independent factor that defines a very major health risk that today is virtually unknown. It probably is the #1 reason so many men still drop dead soon after completing their physical exams with 'flying colors.'

Better Cardiofitness Can Help Most of Our Population

Table 8-4 shows an estimate of a distribution in cardiofitness levels of a population that probably is similar to that of the US population. This sample was taken as an average of two other populations that had an average CFR of 103. About 10% of our population probably has the very high risks of a CFR below 80.

It is likely that genetics can determine at least 10-15% of a person's CFR. Some people that do not exercise and that would have a usual CFR of 90 but also have unfavorable genetics can obtain CFR levels below 80. These persons will be at exceptional risk of suffering major disease.

Table 8-4

Table 8-4: Percentage of Average Population at Levels of the CFR	
CFR Range	**Percent of Population**
Below 70	3
70-79	7
80-89	13
90-99	18
100-109	21
110-119	16
120-129	11
130-139	6
140-149	2
150+	1

Half of our population by definition is at CFR levels below 100. Two hours per week of intensity monitored very brisk walking or a moderate cardio program would provide an important protection for any in this group. A better cardio program could improve CFR by 20 or more. With the exception of perhaps the 20% that now are at good cardiofitness, the entire 80% remainder of our population has a potential of substantially reducing their risk of disease and enjoying a better and longer life by a program of cardio effective exercise.[80]

Today only about 24% of our adult population continues to smoke cigarettes. As mentioned, the fraction of our population that have high cholesterol now can be given statin-type medications. And a variety of medications help control most of those that have high blood pressure.

This analysis shows that improved cardiofitness probably can improve the health and longevity of more people to as large or larger extent than can an improvement in any other major risk factor. And the only known way to improve this risk is adequate cardio-effective exercise.

I hope this will help convince readers and scientists of the major importance of improving and maintaining a good cardiofitness. Getting to a good cardiofitness must be one of the best things I have ever done. If I had not done this I would not be writing this today. With a father that dropped suddenly dead at age 45 and both grandfathers gone by age 61 my family history risk is dismally high. And my calculations say that I probably would have been gone two decades ago if I had not remained cardiofit.

I say once again: Cardiofitness also can make us feel better and more alive nearly every day of a longer and more disease-free life. Improving these other risk factors usually will not develop this very key benefit.

Part Three

The CFR is a Broadly Useful Measure of Cardiofitness

CHAPTER 9

The CFR and What it Means

There are dozens of tests for measuring various aspects of our physical fitness. Some produce results as numbers of how fast we can walk a mile, Others produce arbitrary results only as "Fair," "Good," etc that can be of minimal value. But there has been no single, useful number being widely used that can define quantitatively how cardiofit we are.

A Curious and Near Incredible Fact

Our cardiofitness can be a most important single measure of our present overall health. Yet very few – and this includes most doctors and health professionals – know their level of cardiofitness! A value of total cholesterol may be less than a perfect indicator, but it does give everyone at least some measure of a health risk. The same is true for the two-value method for blood pressure, the number of a fasting glucose and dozens of other direct numerical measures of body condition.

The CFR, or Cardiofitness Ratio, provides this missing measure. It provides a useful single number that defines immediately and simply a level of health and risk. A CFR of 80 immediately shows a man or woman of any age that their cardiofitness is very poor and needs attention. A CFR of 120 shows that they are properly cardiofit for their age. A CFR of 80 means that cardiofitness is 80% of average. A CFR of 120 means that it is 20% above average.

The CFR opens up a fascinating world of information about people that has been virtually buried in dozens of research papers that are long forgotten. I have described the CFR briefly and cited it frequently in previous chapters. I showed that it identified nearly tenfold verified risks of heart disease and up to several-fold risks of other major diseases that were not identified by any other measure. I showed how we need to exercise to improve our CFR level of cardiofitness and reduce our risk. It is appropriate now to tell more about this all important CFR.

Our cardiofitness or CFR – also called cardiovascular fitness, cardiorespiratory fitness or physical fitness – is a physical measure of the capability of our heart and its accompanying cardiovascular system. This system includes thousands of miles of blood vessels that supply the nutrients in blood to all parts of our body. I prefer the word cardiofitness because this is the key subject of our research data. Respiratory fitness is involved but this seven-syllable tongue twister word is not needed.

Incredibly, and as I have shown in the previous chapters, researchers have produced a mass of important research that shows this. But the message about the importance of cardiofitness has not been brought to the public. The CFR provides the missing link that can do this. It is a measure that is simple, meaningful, and can be understood and used by everyone.

The cardiovascular system supplies the oxygen and other nutrients that fuel our body cells. The most respected test of the capability of this system called VO2 Max measures the amount of oxygen that this system can supply when a person is doing maximum possible exercise. The VO2 Max value usually is presented either as liters of oxygen consumed per minute or as this value divided by body weight. This is an expensive test. An approximation of its results usually is obtained by measuring the physical activity level a person can produce when exercising at maximum. An example of this substitute test measures how long a person can stay exercising on a treadmill that has a load that steadily keeps increasing. The values from the approximation tests also are expressed as VO2 Max.

There are three major problems with this VO2 Max measurement. First, it provides an absolute measure that produces different values for men and women of different ages. Thus the numbers produced by the test are of no useful direct meaning to people. Second, the test for this cardiofitness required is not suitable for use by the public. Third, we have no assurance that this maximum type test is really needed for or is a best one for identifying the health value of cardiofitness.

It is unfair to compare the usual VO2 Max of a 60-year-old woman with the twice higher usual value of a young man of age 20. I show in Table 9-1 the published values for the VO2 Max of men and women of different ages having different levels of physical activity. What we really need to know is how our cardiofitness compares with those of our own age and gender. These are the values of concern to us and are values we can understand and improve.

The accepted tests of cardiofitness are far too demanding, expensive and risky to be of general use to people. A dogma exists that this very demanding test has to be used to measure cardiofitness. This has effectively kept cardiofitness

Table 9-1

Table 9-1 Average VO2 Max Values in ml-kg.min for Healthy Active and Sedentary Men and Women vs. Age				
Age	Men		Women	
	Active	Sedentary	Active	Sedentary
20	57.5	48.9	36.7	35.2
30	51.3	44.5	33.5	31.6
40	45.2	40.0	30.4	28.3
50	39.1	35.3	27.3	24.5
60	33.0	31.1	24.2	20.9

from being understood by the vast majority of our population. Millions of people that could have been helped by knowing their cardiofitness risk may already have died prematurely because of this. This dogma may already have shortened the potential lives of millions of people.

The CFR approximates simply the ratio of a person's actual VO2 Max to an average VO2 Max of a person of similar age and gender. We multiply the ratio by 100 to obtain more convenient whole numbers that identify value changes in percents. Researchers usually report changes in cardiofitness of different individuals as percent differences in VO2. The CFR produces these same numbers. But importantly, the CFR not only shows percent changes but identifies an absolute level of cardiofitness that is of major importance to our health. As we shall see, we can approximate our CFR using relatively simple tests that will be acceptable to most people, and that many can use by themselves.

By moving an average value of cardiofitness to 100, we eliminate the need for clumsy massive reference tables to tell us what the various values mean. Without the ratio or CFR basis, a value of cardiofitness would be in fractional non-descriptive numbers that would be virtually useless to people. More about how the CFR was constructed appears in a paper on my website.[60]

The CFR Uniquely Values Both Cardiofitness and Health

The CFR provides both a direct measure of cardiofitness and a direct measure of health. It is the only measure useful to people that does this. The CFR derives first from the results obtained and published by the Cooper

Institute that developed today's most accurate valuation of cardiofitness. It is further supported by results of a dozen other studies relating cardiofitness to risk of heart and other diseases.

The CFR brings the previously disparate results of epidemiology and physiology into a common family for analysis. We have many other different measures of cardiofitness such as a step test, time on a treadmill, times for walking certain distances, and heart rates on an exercise bicycle. None of these other test values has been related directly to risk of major disease and death.

How Cardiofitness Varies for Lifestyle

Average individuals that have been confined to bed rest without any exercise usually develop a CFR of about 70, or 70% of average. The CFR of a typical athlete may range up to 160 to 180. Top athlete Lance Armstrong had an 85 VO2 Max at age 35. This computes to a CFR of 232. New York City Marathon Winner and World Champion Paul Tergat had a 84 VO2 Max at age 37 He also measured 232 CFR. These may be the two of the most cardiofit men in the world. And they probably have an outstanding genetic advantage over most of us. The cardiofitness of most people will measure between values of 80 and 140 CFR.

Table 9-2 provides a panoramic view of how cardiofitness levels vary for individuals doing differing lifestyles. Please try to find the category in this table that corresponds most closely to your likely level of cardiofitness. Some people have a genetic advantage or disadvantage in cardiofitness. Thus some with poor genetics may not reach much above a CFR of 100 even when doing quite a bit of exercise. Others that do rather little exercise may find themselves at a higher level than this table would suggest.

An average person's VO2 Max declines with age partly because of a normal physical decline and partly because of lesser physical activity. The present CFR is designed to reflect only the normal decline of aging, and does not reflect any accompanying effect of reduced physical activity. Thus the CFR of average people will move down somewhat with age because they tend to exercise less as they become older. This decline with age can be stopped and even partly reversed for those that maintain good cardio exercise. An older person can generate a similar increase in cardiofitness as will a younger person from a given exercise amount and intensity.

Table 9-2

LEVELS of CARDIOFITNESS RATIO – or the CFR			
Physical Condition	Usual Exercise	CFR	Physical and Health Indications
Extremely Poor	Prolonged Bed Rest	70	Takes some steps, but not much more than this
Very Poor	Only sitting and Driving, no walking	80	Heart rate movies up rapidly for just one flight of starts
Low Sedentary	Persons of normal activity but doing no planned exercise	90	Heart pounds going up 2 stair flights, walking a mile is distasteful
Avg Sedentary	A few miles of walking each week	100	Can walk fairly briskly, one flight of stairs OK but two is distasteful
Fair Cardiofitness	Two hours per week of brisk walking	110	Can walk fast and up stairs easily.
Good Cardiofitness	Useful moderate cardio exercise for 2 hrs/wk	120	Can walk very fast, jog or run when needed. Move up stairs quickly
Fine Cardiofitness	Programmed good Cardio for 2 hrs/wk	130	Run's up two stair flights, walk, jog or run
Excellent Cardiofitness	Cardio 2 hrs/wk at medium to high heart rates	140	Can work physically long hours, run up multiple flights easily
Usual Athlete	Serious regular cardio at high levels	160	Top physical condition and well being for those
Genetically Gifted Athlete	Maximum Conditioning	170 to 190	Same as above but genetically gifted to reach higher levels
2 of most Fit World Athletes	Maximum Conditioning	232	Extraordinary physical capability and large genetic advantage

The CFR of Populations Over History

During prehistory when most people lived as hunter-gatherers, people probably had quite high levels of cardiofitness. George Mann measured values of 150 CFR for African Masai men that still live this way.[43] A usual CFR of a middle-aged US population probably was 110 to 120 at the turn of the 20th century before the advent of the automobile and when 40% of our population worked on small farms. This estimate derives from cardiofitness measurements in developing country populations because no actual cardiofitness information of that era is available.

The first VO2 Max data published indicated an average of 116 CFR.[61] This was reported by Robinson on a male population of age 50 in Boston in 1938. Rather few people did much planned exercise before about 1970. Before this time most people obtained their cardiofitness from a more active than present lifestyle. Data collected in the US and Europe during the 1960's though the 1980's suggest population average cardiofitness levels at age 50 of about 100 to 105 CFR. These values appear to have been about maintained today. But typical values for those that were selected for exercise research programs as not then exercising were 90 CFR. The population average is higher partly because of the inclusion of some that do good exercise and have CFR levels above 120.

How the CFR Varies with Occupation

Before about 1970 most researchers assumed that cardiofitness from physical activity would depend mostly on the physical activity of occupation. Tests showed the physical activity could be 2,000 calories per day in some heavy physical occupations versus only a few hundred calories per day in light activity occupations. This logical assumption proved to be seriously false. Allard found in Canada that those in heavy physical activity occupations measured only an average of 103 CFR.[62] This was only modestly higher than the CFR of 99 he measured for those in light occupations. This small effect of so much physical activity on cardiofitness seemed surprising.

Another researcher, Gyntelberg of Denmark, found a 103 CFR for those doing heavy physical work and 98 for those doing light work.[63] A study in Norway found a high 125 CFR for lumberjacks that may be the most physically active of occupations. But office workers in Norway had a 115 CFR. My experience in Norway and knowing some of these people suggests that Norwegians are an unusually physical active and athletic people.

Farmers and sharecroppers whose work was very physically active probably developed advantages of 10-20 CFR vs. average. But the majority of individuals in physically active occupations obtained only modestly higher than average values for cardiofitness. The reasons for this have been long known to physiologists. The Heart Theory of Cardiofitness introduced in this book explains quantitatively why calories of occupational physical activity can produce such small improvements in cardiofitness.

Population Distributions of Cardiofitness

Some of the researchers that developed actual values of cardiofitness provided information that could be used to estimate roughly the population distributions of cardiofitness in CFR. Each of these distributions showed a wide likely range in the cardiofitness of individuals compared with an average value. For example, the CFR of individuals in populations that had an average level of cardiofitness close to the US population average of about 100 CFR ranged from below 70 to above 150.

It is useful to compare these distributions of cardiofitness with those due to likely differences in actual exercise. The highest usual confirmed improvements developed in the physiological research were about 25 CFR. This was for exercise of only about a half year. Exercise for a full year should bring this to 30 CFR . Very intensive exercise or very good monitored exercise done over many years could bring improvements due to exercise to 50 CFR or more.

Genetics Can Contribute to Cardiofitness

Even with this as a possible range of cardiofitness likely from exercise, the full range in cardiofitness of individuals in a population may be more than 80 CFR. This still suggests a substantial contribution of genetics to values of the CFR for some individuals in our population. And some of these at the low CFR level could have had extraordinary risks of major disease that now are not identified.

Just as some people have genetically stronger arms and legs than average they also can have more physically capable cardiovascular systems. A paper of the Cooper Institute groups showed that 20% of men and women in the high cardiofitness groups cited no exercise, and some in the low fitness group were doing good exercise.[64] Dr. Samuel Fox noted to me that an occasional robust individual who did little exercise could achieve a good treadmill fitness test result.

My own feeling is that genetics can be responsible for at least a plus or minus ten percent of a measured value of cardiofitness. For example, individuals in a group averaging 90 CFR and doing the same exercise might test from 80 to 100 CFR. Not all of what has been viewed as genetic may be true. For example, people doing little exercise can be obtaining quite different amounts of effective cardio from lifestyle such as how much and how fast they move during a day, and from their occupation and other physical activity they fail to view as exercise.

The Heart Theory of Cardiofitness
Explains the Surprising Results for Occupations

Cardiofitness is a physical measurement of the muscle capability of the heart and its cardiovascular system. The Heart Theory suggests that cardiofitness results from what is resistance exercise of the cardiovascular system. The level of cardiofitness is determined by the highest heart rate and blood flow maintained for about two hours during a week. This result is similar to results from resistance exercise of specific body muscles.

Strength improvement is determined largely by the amount of weight lifted for some determined number of repetitions and time of stress each week. And there is a limiting amount of exercise time such as three exercise sessions per week that can usefully improve muscle. There is a similar limit of about two hours a week of a higher than usual exercise that the cardio muscle can absorb and use. More on this Heart Theory is in Appendix 5 and elsewhere in the book.

Physiologists long have explained the relatively small advantages in cardiofitness and risk of disease for those that worked in very physically active occupations that required many thousands of activity calories each week. Those working all day in occupations conserve their activity and tend to keep heart rates usually below 100 beats per minute. This level of exercise heart rate does not produce cardiofitness effectively. The Master Tables in Appendix 1 show the small improvements on cardiofitness obtained from inadequate exercise heart rates.

The Heart Theory explains further how this happens quantitatively. For example, those in a physically demanding occupation might develop, from thousands of overall physical activity calories, a highest two hours of heart exercise of only 110 beats per minute. This from Master Table 5-2 would produce an increase in cardiofitness of 9 CFR. An otherwise sedentary group doing aerobic dancing at a 120 heart rate for two hours a week would develop a higher CFR of 13 and exert only a few hundred physical activity calories per day.

We do not have the precise figures for actual heart rates maintained during occupations. But the order of magnitude values used in the above example explain easily why occupational physical activity has produced such modest levels as only 103 CFR from thousands of calories per week of physical activity. A person doing far fewer physical activity calories easily could attain CFR values in the 100-110 range from just two hours of quite brisk walking during a week.

Most Research on Physical Activity and Disease Has Been Deficient

Most of the hundred-plus available studies of physical activity and heart disease showed that "physical activity reduces risk." Nearly every study result was heralded as significant and showed that exercise was "good to do." But most studies added very little to our real knowledge.

There were two major problems. First, without the identification of cardiofitness the risk ratios found for best exercise were usually only 1.5 to 2 times. This vastly undervalued the potential of effective cardio exercise. And second, most studies produced little information about what exercises really produced the benefit. Such statistical studies do not tell what people need to do to reduce their risk of disease. This problem was solved by the more meaningful results from research that measured the health value of cardiofitness as shown in Figure 1-1, Table 1-1, Figures 7-1, 7-2 and Appendix 7.

The CFR or Something Like This Seems So Obviously Needed. Why Hasn't it Been Proposed Before?

The answer here is that is was proposed, though under a different name, in my 1982 book on the importance of cardiofitness. Top authority Dr. Samuel Fox, who reviewed the book, found it of appreciable interest and actually proposed the name Heart Performance Index we used for the measure then.

I wrote then and later to various researchers in an attempt to interest them in using it. I encountered the academic equivalent of a solid brick wall. Academic researchers can have little interest in communicating their results to the public. This is true in other fields of science. We recall the publicity about Carl Sagan being looked down on by his peers because he brought astronomy so impressively to the public.

The ultimate effectiveness of health research depends on how much it contributes to benefiting public health. As example, how many people do something different as a result of a research that could contribute to their wellness. Values used by researchers can be too complex for most people to understand without extensive explanation. There is a serious need to convert values used by researchers to values the public can easily understand.

Health Number Values Should Be Designed to Help Doctors and the Public

An example of how researchers failed to communicate well to the public is the use of the Body Mass Index (BMI) for body weight. The present index is really only a statistical factor in metric units that identifies desirable weight by height. Values of about 23.5 for men and women in metric units are most healthful. The actual BMI values would have been much different if they were expressed in English units rather than metric ones. But they would serve the same purpose. The absolute level of the index thus means nothing. The important thing that the BMI reveals is how our weight compares with a healthful weight and how it affects our health.

It would have been incredibly simple to just multiply the present index value in metric units by a factor such as 4.25. With this basis, the BMI of people of healthy weight would be about 100. A BMI value of 150 would show immediately that a person's weight is 50% above healthful. This revelation is both meaningful and disturbing. The values for both weight and the BMI value could have been shown on weight scales. This simple action could have done far more to stimulate people to maintain a healthful weight.

Using the present method a 50% higher weight produces a BMI of 36.3. This is a number that has little useful meaning to people. To understand what it means requires comparison tables that in the real world will rarely ever be conveniently available or used. If the above thought had been given to how the BMI could best help the population, nearly everyone would now know his or her BMI and know what this number means. I have little doubt that many lives could have been lengthened by this simple action. Today the BMI is a near useless number and concept to our population..

We now have an incredible confusion of four numbers on cholesterol for doctors and the public to try to understand: Total cholesterol, HDL cholesterol, LDL cholesterol, and a ratio of Total to HDL cholesterol. I discovered many years ago that the simple chemistry method of using just two measures, total cholesterol and the concentration of HDL in total, would provide a more accurate valuation than using all four numbers. These risk values for total cholesterol and HDL concentration could be easily factored into a single number that identifies more accurately and far more usefully the net health-related result of all those four now needed values. The single concentration value would provide a better valuation for HDL than the two-value present method of a using an absolute value and a ratio.

Can you now quote average, good and poor values for each of the above four measurements of serum cholesterol? Can you interpret the meaning of the different combinations of a total cholesterol, an LDL, an HDL and a total to HDL ratio? I doubt that many can.

The CFR or its equivalent should be endorsed by a large organization that has is seriously interested in helping the public. As for example the American College of Sports Medicine, or the American Heart Association. By using the simple single number and meaningful CFR, we do not need to repeat the failures made in introducing the BMI and cholesterol to the public. A good CFR could be a source of pride. A poor value could stimulate a person's interest in improving it. With availability of simple tests, millions should be tested for their CFR. Nearly everyone will understand immediately what a value of their CFR can mean, and what they may need to do about it. The CFR could become a clearly known and understood number.

The CFR should be of interest to any fitness organization as an introductory measurement that can show clients the need to improve their cardiofitness. The CFR that is directly related to risks of major disease and death can be valuable in demonstrating that exercise programs might provide positive benefits. No other generally useful cardiofitness test can now do this.

Each 3 units of maintained CFR add the equivalent of another year to an average person's healthy life. Knowing their cardiofitness as a single simple understandable number such as the CFR should encourage individuals to exercise and keep exercising.

There Is No Substitute for Knowing Your Actual CFR: This revelation may tell you that you need to move more seriously into a better cardio program. If your CFR is low it will be especially important to avoid poor diets and other high-risk habits. A combination of a low CFR with poor diet and other habits suggest that a person will have a substantially shortened life.

The next chapter shows how a CFR value now can easily be measured

CHAPTER 10

Measuring the Cardiofitness Ratio or the CFR

The two reasons most responsible for the public's present lack of knowledge about cardiofitness have been first, the lack of a clearly identified measure that people could use and understand; and second the lack of a practical accepted test that could be used for measuring it.

The CFR provides the needed measure of cardiofitness. It provides a single number measure to identify cardiovascular health and risk of major diseases. It can show how exercise kind and amount produce their health value. It provides for a coherent organization of the research information on exercise and cardiofitness. It brings results from epidemiology and physiology together into one uniquely useful database. It provides the key measure needed to develop a Global Scientific Analysis of cardiofitness.

This chapter introduces a test most people can take that should provide a useful measure of their CFR. I call it Test C. Two other tests A and B are suggested for those of low cardiofitness.

Many of you do not need to go through this chapter's explanation of the background about cardiofitness tests and the validity of the new test. I describe the actual CFR tests and how to take them in Appendix 2. This convenient section provides all that you need to know to measure your cardiofitness. But I feel that the information that follows here is needed to help convince those involved in testing that we can obtain useful measure of the CFR from some relatively simple specific tests.

The Existing Test for Cardiofitness

Today's accepted test for cardiofitness is the VO2 Max test expressed as ml of oxygen per minute, or this value per kg of body weight. The true basic VO2 Max test measures the actual amount of oxygen a person can consume at maximum exercise. But this test is expensive and involves an assumption that a true maximum physical effort was actually exerted during the test.

A usual VO2 Max substitute test measures a person's workload at an estimated heart rate that is assumed to be that for maximum possible exercise. Another substitute measures the time a person can remain on a treadmill that has a continuously increasing exercise load. A VO2 Max test, usually via substitute, also is used as a medical test by cardiologists to test patients for heart disease. These substitute tests also are expensive and demanding, and involve some participants in a very small risk of a heart attack during the test.

The sanctity of and requirement for the VO2 Max test have been a near religion among many physiologists and related health researchers. This may have been the key has that prevented the vitally important concept of cardiofitness from being provided usefully to our public. A presumed need for this expensive test also has seriously limited the usefulness of much published research on exercise. Because exercise produces most benefits via cardiofitness, research that overlooks this factor can produce only associations that are of minimal scientific or practical value. Most epidemiology researchers have felt that the present VO2 Max test is too expensive and demanding to be included in their studies.

There are problems with tests for the VO2 Max. It is difficult to know if a person is really exercising to maximum. A substitute test often exercises individuals to near maximum and then extrapolates result to a workload at a computed maximum heart rate. This estimated maximum heart rate can be an inaccurate number. An actual maximum heart rate at 5% to 95% limits can vary over a range of more than 30 beats per minute.

I have included more on this problem in Appendix 4. It can be argued that when this estimated value of heart rate is used rather than an actual maximum, the VO2 Max substitute test is no longer a true VO2 Max test but a type of sub-maximal test performed at high heart rates.

About Cardiofitness Tests

The actual maximum heart rate test should provide a best index of athletic performance, as this recognizes a value at actual heart rate rather than some formula for maximum heart rate. And this may have been one reason for the long-time preference of experts for the maximum test over submaximal tests. But this reason does not necessarily apply for a cardiofitness test that measures risk of disease. More on this follows.

What Cardiofitness Test is Best for Measuring Risk of Disease?

Arraiz obtained a similar risk level for heart disease from a simple step test that others obtained using more expensive VO2 Max tests.[7] This and other evidence we have suggest that results from almost any kind of a cardiofitness test probably would be useful for estimating the cardiofitness that is related to risk of disease.

The outstanding relationship of risk of heart disease vs. the CFR shown in Figure 9-1 was obtained from VO2 estimates developed from a variety of cardiofitness tests. None really was a true maximal test. Most were taken at high exercise heart rates, but one was taken at much lower than maximum heart rates. At this writing there is no evidence that a particular cardiofitness test as sub-maximal or maximal or other is better for identifying the risk of disease.

A problem here is the low regard that been placed on the word 'sub-maximal.' It has been claimed that results of a fitness tests at lower than maximal heart rates do not correlate well with results of maximal heart rate tests. This presumably makes such tests 'no good.' A researcher could risk having his research paper rejected if he did not develop cardiofitness using the approved maximum type tests.

This belief has essentially forced the use of very high exercise heart rate tests for measuring cardiofitness that are difficult and expensive. This in turn has kept the importance of cardiofitness away from the public. And this in turn probably has shortened uncounted millions of people's lives.

There are reasons why those older sub-maximum cardiofitness test results did not correlate well with those taken at maximum rate. Results from the largest-yet database of cardiofitness now show that useful values of cardiofitness can be obtained from sub-maximal test measurements.

What Does a Cardiofitness Test Really Measure?

All cardiofitness tests measure a physical capability of the cardiovascular system to move blood and oxygen. Actually, this muscle capability of the cardio system per se may not be the truly casual factor that produces the health benefits of cardiofitness.

In order to create and maintain cardio muscle the heart has to 'train' by beating faster and moving more blood than usual for some time. That faster beating produces a higher blood flow throughout the cardiovascular system that opens up arteries as in shown by the remarkable photos in Figure 7-3 of Chapter 7. This faster beating also circulates dozens of potentially useful nutrients, including oxygen, throughout thousands of miles of arteries, veins and capillaries. I visualize this improved circulation as a likely major casual mechanism by which physical activity produces the cardiofitness that protects from heart and so many other diseases.

If we accept this, the muscle capability of the cardiovascular system becomes a useful factor of statistical association. This muscle capability provides a measure of the amount of the higher blood circulation that must be periodically occurring to develop and maintain a particular level cardiofitness.

A cardiofitness test most appropriate thus should be one that tests fitness and blood flow at the actual highest levels of exercise used by individuals. There would be no purpose for using a test done at the much higher maximum rates that are never actually used.

In summary, I see no cogent scientifically-based reason why an expensive maximum level test for cardiofitness should be a need for measuring the cardiofitness level for identifying a risk of health. Further, we do have a test that is done at usual sub-maximal exercise heart rates and that actually does forecast accurately the result obtained at estimated maximum heart rates.

The Cooper Institute Cardiofitness Tests

We now have an outstanding basis for development of the needed cardiofitness test. This is the more the 21,000 actual maximum cardiofitness tests developed by the Cooper Institute group during their research project. Results from these tests have been extensively published in detail. The size and significance of this database dwarfs any other that now exists. And it seems unlikely that any other database approaching this one will be developed in the foreseeable future.

Importantly and as I showed before, the researchers showed that results of this database are directly related to risks of heart disease, cancer, and all causes of death. Thus use of the Cooper Institute database provides for cross-linking cardiofitness levels and health results of men and women of ages 20 to well past 60 having all grade levels of cardiofitness.

The Balke Fitness test used in the Cooper research exercised persons walking at 3.3 miles per hour on a treadmill starting at zero grade. Grade was at 2% the second minute, with an increase in test incline each further minute of 1%. Thus at 5 minutes the incline was 5%, at 10 minutes it was 10%, and at 15 minutes it was 15%. A user's cardiofitness was graded as time spent on the treadmill until a participant had to give up walking on it any longer. A participant's heart rate increased steadily during the test from an initial resting value to a level near or at maximum at the end of the test.

This unique data-base provides values of participants heart rates at 5, 10, and 15 minutes into the test together with the measured values of VO2 Max. This provided a direct basis for testing how well the sub-maximal or lower heart rates during the test correlated with the final results of VO2 Max and CFR. No other database exists today that provides even a small fraction of the information developed from these 21,000 cardiofitness tests.

The heart rates measured at each time, say 5 minutes into the test, changed substantially with the level of cardiofitness measured. For example, the low-fitness group of men had 5-minute heart rates averaging about 135; the middle fitness group of men had rates had 5-minute heart rates of 115, and the high fitness group had 5-minute heart rates of only 105. Women of different levels of cardiofitness also had similarly large differences in the heart rates at the 5-minute time into the tests.

When analyzed with more sophisticated mathematics I found the group average heart rates taken at 5 minutes into the tests actually forecast both the final group average VO2 Max and CFR values almost exactly.

I have posted in the reference on my website the actual formulas derived and much more about this analysis.[60] For the CFR, the correlation for men is 99%, and for women 99%. For the VO2 Max the correlation was 99% and 99%. Most values of the average VO2 Max values on groups were forecast from the 5-minute heart rate within one unit of VO2 Max. Most values of the CFR are forecast within about 2 units.

What This Means is Exciting

We do not have to develop a costly and demanding maximum test to measure our cardiofitness. We can get a good estimate of this value from a far more simple test done in five minutes. The 5-minute heart rate forecast the CFR directly with no further effect of user age needed. A forecast of VO2 Max from the 5-minute rate did require a substantial modifier for user age.

This extensive data-base included results for both men and women of ages from 20 to well past 60 having cardiofitness levels from 80 to above 140. This represents a demographic of a large majority of the US population. And finally, this test not only does forecast VO2 Max values but also measures cardiofitness at levels that may be more accurate for estimating the risk of major disease.

This forecast of VO2 Max should not be surprising. It is well known that after some modest elevation above its resting rate, the heart moves the same quantity of blood with each added beat. Thus we should expect to obtain the same result for tests at differing heart rates. I found the same near perfect but no better correlations of heart rates taken at 10 and 15 minutes into the maximal test with the final test values of VO2 Max and CFR. Thus it seems likely that we do not need to obtain results at the very high heart rates in tests that can require 30 or more minutes and the far more demanding exercise needed to reach a full maximum effort.

This New Finding Confronts Heresy

If I have read this once I must have read it a hundred times: "Sub-maximum fitness tests do not forecast maximum test results well." But where is the real evidence on this? I looked for useful evidence but simply could not find it. It seems to be one of those things that gain acceptance from endless repetition. Recall that every health expert knew that exercise was bad for heart health back in 1950. And that they all knew that calories of all foods had exactly the same effect on body weight before Atkins challenged this idea.

There are good reasons why poor correlations of fitness tests could have been found in the past. A direct correlation between a sub-maximal test result and a VO2 Max result is impossible. This is because a maximum heart rate declines at a much faster rate than does a sub-maximal heart rate with increase in a person's age. And without including an effect of age in the equation, the heart rate at five minutes cannot correlate with the VO2 Max final result. Also, a true maximum test will use a true measured heart rate that can be quite different than one from a formula that is involved in using a sub-maximal test.

Finally, there is that previously noted consideration. There are good reasons to believe that the best cardiofitness test for risk of disease should be done at the actual higher heart rates obtained in exercise. The VO2 Max test is more useful for assessing athletic performance. The proposed CFR tests should be more useful for measuring the risk of major disease.

Moving to a Practical and Useful Cardiofitness Test

We have the evidence that we can obtain a good estimate of cardiofitness from the 5-minute result in the Cooper-Balke test method. A direct replication of the this test would require increasing heart rate each minute for 5 minutes to get a result.

But this detail probably is not needed. Experience in fitness testing shows that user heart rates plateau after being exposed to a given energy load for about 3 minutes. This means that starting the test at the treadmill speed of 3.3 miles per hour at an incline of 5% and continuing to walk on it at this rate for 3 minutes should produce the same or very similar heart rates to that produced in the Cooper-Balke 5-minute test.

This is a very simple test that most people that do exercise can take. The test involves setting the treadmill at 3.3 mph and a 5% incline, walking on it for 3 minutes and then measuring the exercise heart rate. It could be possible to start the test at lower speed for the first minute and work up to the full 3.3 mph slowly. This heart rate obtained translates directly into CFR values from separate tables for men and women. I call this test "Cardiofitness Test C."

It is vitally important that you start any cardiofitness testing with appropriate care because any fitness test can be too demanding for some people. Please follow carefully the suggestions in Appendix 2.

This or any other cardiofitness test will be taken best with the aid of an exercise facility expert in a monitored facility or a personal trainer. A person that has not exercised regularly should be approved for it by a doctor before doing this test. Test C may be too strenuous for many women and for some men having low cardiofitness. Alternate cardiofitness Tests A and B done at lower exercise levels are suggested in Appendix 2 for those of low cardiofitness.

But after careful reading and observing the cautions noted, the test probably can be taken easily by many individuals that perform cardio exercise regularly. It can be exciting for people to learn how their cardiofitness in the

CFR that is directly related to health improves as they continue exercise.

The Life Ahead Computer program provided as a free download will compute the CFR from heart rates taken in this proposed cardiofitness Test C. The program also will roughly estimate CFR values from two different less strenuous treadmill fitness tests A and B. Life Ahead also will develop values of the CFR from results of the Bruce treadmill method, from results of exercise bicycle tests, and from a VO2 Max measurement. The program also will estimate CFR values from lifestyle and from wide variety of exercise amounts and intensities. More on this is in Appendix 6.

A comparison of CFR estimated from exercise with that computed from an actual test will provide a measure of cardiofitness genetic susceptibility. Simple formulas are provided for translating values of the CFR to VO2 Max.

Weight and the CFR

Before leaving this chapter, I should address the problem of body weight and cardiofitness. Results from the primary VO2 Max test are expressed as liters of oxygen consumed per minute. This includes no modifier for weight. An alternate is to divide this by body weight. Research results usually are expressed via one or both of these measures and there is no certainty as to which is more meaningful. For athletics the weight adjustment seems logical as a heavier person will require a higher oxygen consumption level to run uphill at a given speed. But this does not apply for a forecast of a risk of disease. Heart attacks are not usually caused by a maximum level of exercise. They occur at all levels of physical activity, including sleep.

There is no scientific basis for using an adjustment for body weight in the VO2 Max method. A weight adjustment assumes that a person who loses weight via diet but does not exercise will obtain an improvement in cardiofitness. This seems unlikely because a loss in weight does not change directly the capability of the cardiovascular system to pump blood. A highest usual blood flow rate in the cardiovascular system is the key that protects against disease.

The use of a proportional weight adjustment is thus not appropriate in a measure of cardiofitness. The present CFR derives for men and women of average size and weight. There probably will be some bias in the health valuation of persons at a given CFR that differ much in size or weight from this average. But at this time no valid way for including this factor is known. Being overweight should be segregated as a visible specific and independent health factor, as for example in the BMI, and should not be included further in the CFR. Attempting to recognize an effect of weight in two different risk factors could cause serious confusion.

Should We Wait?

It would be desirable to have a cardiofitness test that is endorsed by some respected medical organization. But let us face the reality of how long it takes to accomplish something like this. A really useful cardiofitness test for people that identifies health has not been revealed in the past 25 years of need. It may or may not happen in the remaining lifetime of millions that could benefit from it.

I am convinced that nearly any kind of a cardiofitness test could supply the present need for a useful test of cardiofitness. But this Test C is the only test basis that is clearly shown with high significance to be related both to cardiofitness and to risk of disease and death. It derives directly on the largest study of its kind. Why not use it? The test is based on a far larger body of research data than is any other cardiofitness test.

Those experienced in treadmill testing may prefer to duplicate the first five minutes of the exact Cooper-Balke test rather than use the alternate I suggest. Some may prefer to try both tests to assure that they produce near similar results. But increasing the load each minute, as needed in the Cooper-Balke test, involves a requirement that may need expert assistance.

I hope many groups and organizations will try using these tests and report their results so that we can get experience with them soon. We need good research on results of these tests. I will welcome any comments and results from those that use any of these proposed cardiofitness tests

Bringing Cardiofitness to Medicine

Cardiofitness is a largely independent health risk factor of major importance to health and life. A cardiofitness measurement deserves inclusion in usual medical examinations as an important risk of health that today is overlooked.

The 3-minute test proposed here could be a central test basis for this purpose. But because many people will be in very poor physical condition, a test system should start at lower intensity to keep heart rates within a conservative range. There should be test alternates for those that cannot walk or have other physical problems. Any development of a cardiofitness test should recognize clearly that this test should be useable in a physician's office and it should not be costly or difficult to take.

A suitable test for medicine will start at a very low intensity level and increase each half or full minute. Heart rate will be monitored, and a test result used when heart rate reaches some moderate predetermined level. A CFR could be computed at any test load. A level of Test C would be the standard and final test for those that can reach this level. CFR values at other test levels can be related to and derived for the results of tests at lower stress levels. The test should be completed in maximum of five minutes or lesser time.

We Do Not Need Researcher Type Measures

The standard approach to testing in the health area will be to try to teach the public to use conventional researcher values that for cardiofitness are VO2 Max and Mets. I cited the problems with cholesterol and the BMI when using researcher type values directly rather than modifying them to equivalent values designed to better help doctors and the public.

This same confusion can be produced again by using such complex research measures that are not useful without extensive comparison tables. The values produced will be of no use to the public without adjustment. The CFR that directly provides the useful age and gender adjusted values of cardiofitness level that are immediately meaningful. This in turn will provide by far the greatest contribution to the public health.

A well implemented and designed exercise program should improve CFR by from 10% to 20% after a year of exercise. An individual will need values of measured cardiofitness from multiple tests having a reproducibility of 1 to 2 CFR to determine progress in improving fitness toward such goals.

The CFR together with the multiple use of the proposed cardiofitness tests will supply this need. To obtain the equivalent of an age adjusted value such as the CFR from Mets or VO2 for measuring health risk, reference tables must be developed in a matrix of at least eighty age segments and by 50 cardiofitness segments for each gender. Such large tables will be difficult to work with. I see no useful purpose in providing such research values and tables for adjustment to the public.

Part Four

Exercise and Cardiofitness:

Mythology and Fact

CHAPTER 11

CARDIOFITNESS HELPS REDUCE WEIGHT

Many people and perhaps most women exercise to reduce their weight than to improve their long range health. People starting a program to reduce weight often start by walking more. This is certainly a good thing to do. But sadly, doing just this usual kind of walking may do little to reduce their weight.

Reducing Weight by Exercise Is Difficult

Exercising to reduce weight can be ineffective when compared with reducing calories from diet. The more accurate data I will show suggest that one hour of walking at 2.5 miles per hour pace will burn only about 100 calories. This only one-third of the 300 calorie burn often incorrectly cited for walking in books and on the internet. It takes 3500 fewer calories to lose a pound in weight.

This means that it will take 35 hours of such walking to lose just one pound. Thus if you walk at this pace the two hours per week needed for best improvement in health, it will take about 17 weeks to contribute a miserly one-pound reduction in weight.

A single portion of some presumed healthful foods can offset a 100 calorie reduction from walking. Consider a banana at 105 calories; a half cantaloupe at 90 calories or a slice of cheese at 110 calories. A small 3-oz portion of steak at 250 calories, or 3-oz of chicken leg at 170 calories will add even more to weight.

Thus if diet is not strictly reduced and carefully monitored, ordinary walking will do little to reduce your weight. It is just too easy to eat up the usual small benefit obtained from exercise.

Published Values for Exercise Calories Can Be Misleading

There are a vast number of incorrect calorie values in diet books and on the internet about how exercise burns calories. These values are misleading for two reasons. First, they usually include the calories of basal metabolism needed to keep the body warm and alive. Those calories that are burned just sitting in a chair are not due to our exercise. Second, these values often do not recognize how energy calories develop from intensity of exercise.

There are two kinds of physical activity calories: Total Calories and Net Calories. Total Calories are what researchers measure. Total calories include the calories of our exercise plus the metabolic calories that we would consume without any exercise. Net calories represent the Total Calories minus the metabolic calories that we would burn even if we did not do any exercise. Net Calories are what we really derive from our exercise.

Figure 11-1 shows the actual calories needed for walking different speeds in kilometers and miles per hour for 150-pound persons. This now classic scientific research information published by Passmore and Durnin was developed by five different researchers that obtained nearly identical results.[65] This shows Net energy calories per hour at the outside left, and Total energy calories per minute at the inside left. The scale at bottom show miles per hour and kilometers per hour pace. Note first that the curved line in Figure 11-1 starts on the left scale at just below the 2 total energy calories per minute for zero miles per hour of walking. This shows about 100 calories per hour at zero miles per hour.

The amount for zero or no walking is the usual energy needed just for basal metabolism. These calories are burned when not doing any exercise. Note also how the line fitting the data curves sharply upward to recognize the many more calories burned at higher walking speeds.

The legends inside the chart are for pace and Total Calories per minute. I have shown outside of the outer lines the walking pace in miles per hour and the Net Calorie per hour values. The cross hatch lines in the graph are for these Net calories. For walking at 5 miles per hour these values move up to 400 Net Calories per hour of exercise vs. the only 100 Net calories per hour at 2.5 miles per hour.

Note the very large effect of walking pace. Walking 2 hours at a com-

Figure 11-1

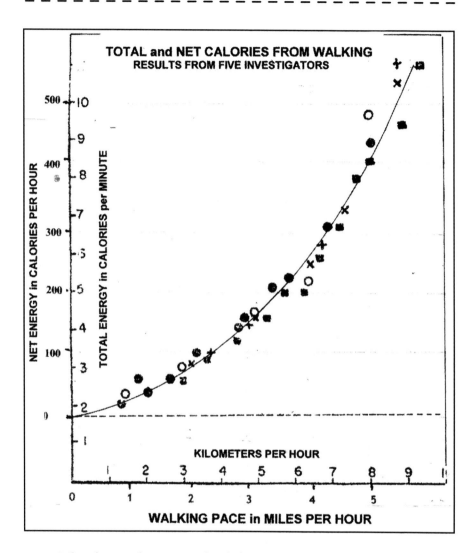

mon 2.5 miles per hour pace develops only 200 calories. Walking at 4.5 miles per hour triples this to 620 calories. You get the same calorie benefit for increasing pace at 2 hours per week as for walking 6 hours at a normal pace. You can multiply these values by the ratio of your weight to 150 for better accuracy.

Getting Calories from Exercise:

A useful reduction in weight by exercise requires a substantial level of exercise intensity. Average pace walking takes far too much time to be effective. To make some progress in weight reduction you need to target at least 250 calories per hour of exercise. This in turn requires brisk walking in the 4 to 4.5 mile per hour range. Even this takes off only an estimated one pound each seven weeks. You probably will get somewhat more calories from exercise than these values due to calorie after-burn that is discussed later. Reducing weight by usual levels of exercise will be unsuccessful unless it is accompanied by strict diet control.

Another method for estimating your direct exercise calories from any kind of exercise is to use your exercise heart rate. Recall how heart rate elevation produced cardiofitness. This same elevation of heart rate above our low resting heart rate is the engine of the body that produces cardiofitness. And this same heart engine is the one that consumes calories of energy. Thus the higher your heart rate elevation, the higher the number of direct calories burned.

Table 11-2

Net Energy Calories and Heart Rate Elevations above Resting Rate				
Low Resting Heart Rate	**50**	**60**	**70**	**80**
Heart Rate Elevation per Minute				
40	160	135	115	100
50	250	210	180	160
60	360	300	260	230
70	490	410	350	310
80	640	540	460	400
90	815	680	580	510

Table 11-2 shows the calories usually required to support various heart rate elevations above its resting rate. Results are shown at the four different resting heart rates used for the Master Tables of cardiofitness development. The values in the left column are heart rate elevations, not exercise heart rates. To obtain an elevation, subtract your resting heart rate from your exercise heart rate.

128

As example, suppose your resting heart rate is 70 beats per minute. If you exercise aerobically at say a 120 heart rate, your elevation is 120 minutes, 70 or 50 beats per minute. For the low resting rate column of 70 this will produce a calorie burn of 180 per hour of exercise. Moving your heart rate to 140 would be a 70 elevation, and this would burn a twice higher 350 calories per minute. Energy demand thus moves up sharply with aerobic exercise heart rate. Again, these values all are for average persons weighing 150 pounds.

Table 11-2 shows that the intensities of exercise that produce cardiofitness best also improve calorie burn best. As cardiofitness improves and resting heart rate moves lower, you can develop more effective exercise calories when exercising at the same heart rate. The same higher heart rate elevation that produces cardiofitness effectively also increases energy calories most effectively.

Aerobic or Resistance Exercise: Which is Better for Reducing Weight?

The arguments about this can be fierce among proponents of these alternate forms of exercise. Reading some of these arguments could relate the myth that doing one could produce a large difference in your weight. This is wrong.

The tables I have used and others on the internet suggest typical values in the order of 400 total and 300 net calories per hour of direct burn from usual weight lifting or resistance exercises. This compares with the calories of fairly fast walking. Vigorous running can produce a burn of up to a twice higher 800 calories per hour. Based just on these actual measurements, high level aerobic exercise usually will consume substantially more direct calories during the time of exercise than will resistance exercise during actual times of exercise. But this is just the start of the story.

Resistance exercise can involve only about 10-12 minutes of actual exercise stress during a session. Substantial time is spent resting. Thus heart rates can move up rapidly during lifting weights but drop down during the intervening periods. Thus the usual direct burn calories from Table 11-2 above for resistance exercise would be rather low.

A first problem is that of calorie after-burn. All exercise derives part of its energy from body chemical stores of glycogen. Resistance exercise derives most of its energy by depleting these stores. This depletion is then restored by a modestly higher heart rate for 12 or more hours. See Figure 4-1 in Chapter 4 for as an example of calorie after-burn. Resistance exercise derives much more of its energy from these chemical stores than does aerobic exercise. This larger after-burn offsets at least partly offsets the higher direct burn advantage of aerobic exercise.

Another factor is that muscle building is better from resistance exercise, and that body muscle will burn more calories after it is formed from an improved metabolic rate. Some early claims about this contended that muscle increases this burn by 50 or more calories per day per pound. These value are now rejected because more correct values measured appear to be in the range of 6-15 calories per day per pound of muscle formed.

If we take the higher above value of 15, this represents a calorie burn of 105 calories per week per pound of muscle. For 3 pounds of muscle added from 10 weeks of vigorous resistance training, this would burn 315 calories per week. This adds a quite significant 50% to the direct calorie burn in three 40-minute resistance exercise sessions per week of perhaps 600 net calories per week. One study showed that resistance exercise did produce about three times as much muscle as did aerobic exercise. If we accept this, good resistance exercise might burn about 200 more calories per week than will moderate level aerobic exercise of two hours per week. This offsets still more of the higher direct calories burn of aerobic exercise.

But muscle weighs more than the fat it replaces, and this part of the advantage for building muscle from resistance exercise could be lost when measured on the weight scale. A response here is that a person's figure will be improved a bit despite this problem of muscle weighing more than fat. But this complicates the problem a bit more.

As another consideration, two studies I could find that directly compared results for similar amounts of resistance and aerobic exercise suggested that the two types of exercise were about equally effective in reducing body fat.[76,77] Finally, we have the difficult problem of measuring and comparing accurately how vigorously each type of exercise is done.

The evidence we have suggests that each kind of exercise done with similar intensity should help produce slow, modest and near similar reductions in weight. It is doubtful that any practical research will be able to answer absolutely the difficult question of whether aerobic or resistance exercise is better for weight control. But this question of "Which type of exercise reduces weight the more" becomes of lesser consequence when we consider how exercise should be programmed for best contribution to overall health and life. More on this follows

Obtaining Weight Reduction from Exercise

The BIG thing that can reduce weight is diet. Any difference in calorie burn for usual different kinds of exercise can be small when compared to potential weight differences from changes in diet.

Wayne Westcott of the Quincy, Massachusetts YMCA reported results of a very large population of 1,644 men and women that did 10 weeks of monitored resistance and aerobic exercise, presumably without any accompanying diet program. Those that performed two weekly sessions of resistance training obtained no loss in body weight. Those performing three weekly sessions of resistance training obtained a insignificant loss of a.1.3 pounds. The overall actual average weight loss of the 1,644 people was an insignificant 0.6 pounds.

If we calculate from the calorie burn what the weight loss should have been, we come up with a value of 3 to 4 pounds. Yet they only lost an insignificant 0.6 pounds!

It seems clear that those who exercised simply ate up much of their potential weight benefit. Drastic differences in exercise such as from military training or similar serious physical activity can produce substantial reductions in weight. But these are not the usual types of programs used to reduce their weight. Without strict attention to diet control, acceptable exercise may do little to reduce weight.

Cardiofitness Can Help

Table 11-1 above suggests you need to walk at 3.5 to 4.5 miles per hour to reduce weight effectively. Paradoxically, you may not be able to walk this fast if you are not cardiofit. Table 11-2 shows this reality. Thus to lose weight effectively by exercise you really need to become cardiofit. It is not what you do but how vigorously you do it that burns calories. This applies not just to walking but to all other types of exercise.

You may be able to nearly double your benefit of exercise in reducing weight by moving your walking pace higher. A similar thing happens in resistance exercise. As you become stronger you will be lifting more weight with each exercise. And as you lift more weight you will burn more calories.

CHAPTER 12

Resistance Exercise and Health

There has been an explosion of interest during the past two decades in resistance exercise. This is the exercise that involves strengthening the arms, legs, and other body muscles. The publicity that exercise is "Good" for health implies that resistance exercise also must be good for health. Exercise trainers today are promoting resistance exercise as a health measure. This is sometimes proposed as an alternate to aerobic exercise. We now even have some overzealous bodybuilders claiming that "Resistance exercise is all you need to do." It is useful thus to review what the available research actually tells us.

The new Heart Theory shows that cardio exercise improves the heart and its cardiovascular system from a type of resistance exercise. Cardio exercise occupies a unique position in the hierarchy of muscle training. The cardio system can be trained only by training some other body muscle that in turn makes the heart beat faster. Thus all exercise trains both some specific body muscle and the cardio muscle.

But most cardio exercise trains only the legs. Swimming trains mostly the arms. We can visualize a theoretically optimum exercise that trains all body muscles simultaneously and sufficiently while also producing the needed training of the cardio system. This will produce an optimum results in a minimum of needed exercise time.

Resistance exercise usually involves 8–10 exercises to include the major muscle groups of chest, shoulders, arms, back, abdomen, thighs and lower legs. Using 1 RM as a maximum weight that can be lifted, 30–40% of this weight for upper body and 50–60% of this weight for lower body should be lifted for a minimum of 8–10 repetitions. When 12–15 repetitions can be lifted, weight should be increased. Each series of repetitions is called a set. A typical workout should be done on 2–3 non-consecutive days each week, with 2 days as a minimum. Exercises for flexibility of key muscles should be included.

Health Benefits from Resistance Training

Resistance training usually trains a much wider variety of body muscles than does aerobic exercise. I have long sought to find reasons supporting the health benefits of resistance exercise. Randy Braith and Kerry Steward of the University of Florida published in 2006 a substantial review of 104 studies of resistance exercise training and its role in preventing cardiovascular disease.[66] This review confirmed that resistance training produces many of the same benefits shown for aerobic exercise. These include:

- Reduces body weight.
- Improves body density and reduces risk of osteoporosis
- Decreases incidence of injuries and risk of falls.
- Reduces blood pressure
- Reduces arthritic pain
- Improves glucose tolerance
- Improves values of cholesterol

But beyond these benefits for all exercise, resistance exercise might add to that of aerobic exercise:

- Improves risk of osteoporosis further by protecting more bones and protecting them better
- Can improve appearance and body image better
- Improves performance in more sports and recreation
- Increases body strength further for daily living
- Improves flexibility of a more extensive number of body joints
- Reduces pain from arthritis
- Increases muscle mass and body metabolism better

133

Quantifying Health Benefits from Exercises

The key problem is that most conventional resistance exercises do not usefully improve cardiofitness. The short term bursts of energy required in usual resistance-type exercise do not increase heart rate nearly as effectively as does longer term aerobic-type exercise. It usually takes about 3 minutes of steady exercise for a heart rate to increase to its highest, or plateau level, rate. A maintained exercise heart rate and heart rate elevation over time is required to produce cardiofitness. Nearly every study of cardiofitness during the past four decades, starting with Kenneth Cooper's research in the 1960's, has shown from zero to rather small improvement in cardiofitness or likely reduction in risk of disease from conventional resistance training.

I showed in Chapter 7 that perhaps 85% of the potential health benefits from aerobic exercise are due to improved cardiofitness which is a primary need to protect against cardiovascular diseases and cancer. I tried but could not verify objectively any further useful reductions in risk of major disease for the above factors that are improved best by resistance training. There must be some benefits but they appear to be small.

A Health Professionals Study did find a modest 35% reduction in risk of heart disease for men doing weight training from what was not a direct study.[26] This beneft probably is high because many people doing weight training exercise also do some aerobic exercise on machines such as treadmills and bicycles. It is not possible to separate out such benefits accurately by usual statistical methods. But using the scale that assigns 85% of health benefit to aerobic exercise, it will be difficult to verify more than perhaps 15 to 20% of this health benefit to accompanying resistance exercise.

There are benefits from resistance training that we cannot quantify. There is the joy of having a more fit body. The added arm strength for use in life can be satisfying. Flexibility can be improved further and this can prevent some very troubling problems in later life. But most of these advantages also can accrue from aerobic exercise.

Many people today are working out faithfully in the gym. But even a major body-building program may not produce the cardio exercise needed for health. Unless exercisers also do accompanying and adequate aerobic exercise, they may not be doing very much to improve their health.

But there is another way. This is to do resistance exercise that simultaneously improves cardiofitness. More on this follows.

Times Needed for Exercise

A major problem that faces most people today is the time required for exercise. Proponents of exercise seem to have little regard for the amount of time they ask people to devote. We have had official proposals for doing an hour a day of walking and others for doing three hourly sessions each week of resistance exercise. Add to this ten hours, the time of getting to facilities, dressing, warm-up and cool-down and we can have little time left to do anything else.

Research now verifies that we can obtain maximum aerobic benefits from just two hours of exercise each week. The available research shows that 3 weekly sessions of resistance exercise develop only small benefits beyond 2 sessions per week. A minimum time for supplementary resistance exercise thus could be 30 minutes for each of two sessions per week. This assumes that facilities for doing both types of exercise are available at the same location, as in a gym or at home. This gives us a total of 3 hours per week needed for proper exercise.

If this is an acceptable time to you, fine. By allocating a full three hours each week for exercise you will have widely available alternates for scheduling. But three hours per week still is a demand many busy working people will not accept. It should be possible to develop both useful resistance exercise and adequate aerobic exercise within or mostly within this same two hour per week time frame. To accomplish this, resistance and flexibility training also must be done in a way that can produce heart rate elevations of at least 40 to 50 beats per minute above low resting heart rates. The fact that most past resistance training programs have produced little gains in cardiofitness suggests that most of these programs have not produced adequate exercise heart rates.

Improving Cardio Benefits from Resistance Exercise

The idea of combining aerobic and resistance training is not new. A so-called circuit resistance training protocol includes lifting lighter weights with shorter rest periods between exercises. Moving faster between exercises and using higher numbers of repetitions circuit training introduces a better aerobic component into resistance training. The objective is to obtain continuous elevations in heart rate from different modes of resistance exercise.

Another approach is to keep heart rate elevated by switching from shorter aerobic sessions on a treadmill to high repetition resistance exercises. The times during which heart rate elevations of 40 to 50 beats per minute are developed in resistance training can be subtracted from the two-hour time needed for best aerobic exercise. If all resistance exercise can be performed at such elevated heart rates, it should be theoretically possible to develop adequate benefits from both kinds of exercise within the two-hour total period needed for best benefits from aerobic exercise.

Combined Benefits of Aerobic and Resistance Training Are Being Achieved

Many exercise programs attempt to combine aerobic and resistance training. The now popular Curves program for women uses a type of circuit resistance training. Women exercise on about a dozen different hydraulic machines that develop increased heart rates for cardio while at the same time training a variety of other body muscles. This program has the potential of providing useful resistance and aerobic training in just two hours each week. The results depend on how seriously women use the program. Those who use it tepidly or as a social get-together get little benefit. I comment more about this interesting program in a following chapter.

A study of combined aerobic and resistance training by Takeshima developed for eighteen 68-year-old men and women developed a very high 29% increase in CFR and useful muscular strength increases of knee, back, chest, and shoulder.[69] This increase in CFR would produce a very large reduction in risks of major disease. This confirms that it is possible to obtain good cardiofitness benefits from specially-designed combined aerobic and resistance exercise.

The Need for Combination Aerobic-Resistance Exercise Programs for Men

Popular programs providing monitored heart rates are now mostly used by women. Many and perhaps most men today develop their own personal exercise programs without help of any advice on desirable exercise heart rates and times of exercise. Many men exercise in gyms and obtain inadequate cardio-type exercise. Others do cardio but no resistance exercise. The guides in this book about exercise heart rates via the Master Tables and the need for time of exercise should be helpful to both men and women in developing their own programs. But still it will not be easy for individuals to develop a combination aerobic-resistance exercise program that can save substantial amounts exercise time.

A program that will develop combinations of heart-rate-monitored aerobic and resistance exercise at perhaps two levels of exercise intensity could provide a substantial benefit to men. I visualize this program as being different than that of Curves in the use of specific exercises and format, but providing a substantial help to men that wish to start exercise or improve their present programs.

Three 40-minute sessions each week or even four 30-minute sessions should provide needed exercise to reach the Good Goal for cardiofitness and at the same time develop the important needs for other body strength and flexibility now usually developed in resistance training. Three 40-minute sessions could be could be scheduled on the alternate days that appear to be most effective for training.

Reducing Exercise Time by Combined Exercises

The Heart Theory of cardiofitness shows that cardiofitness develops from the increase in heart rate elevation above resting rate maintained for up to 2 hours per week. The research suggests that the first hour may contribute nearly 60% and 1½ hours of exercise might contribute 86% of that for the total two hours of exercise.

It seems reasonable that if a resistance program is added to an aerobic program, the time for aerobic exercise could be reduced. For example, if moderate improvements in exercise heart rates are improved in the resistance training, we could reduce the aerobic component to 1½ hours per week. If heart rate elevations in resistance training are improved to the 110 to 120 beat per minute aerobic level, a combined program approaching only two hours per week could be developed.

The expected improvement in cardiofitness from any resistance exercise session can be estimated from the Master Tables in Appendix 1. We need only the average heart rate elevation above its resting rate and time of exercise to do this. An average exercise heart rate could be obtained using recording heart rate monitors. This will make exploration of cardio benefits from resistance exercise far easier than having to run actual cardiofitness test data on every possibility. Such monitored exercise heart rates could show clearly why resistance exercise has failed to produce needed cardiofitness health benefits. This should point the way toward methods for improving the cardio health benefits from resistance exercise.

CHAPTER 13

HEART RATES IN LIVING AND IN EXERCISE

Exercise heart rate is the key factor that develops cardiofitness. Yet most people pay little attention to how their heart beats. Before about 1995 exercise heart rates were extensively promoted as a guide to exercise. But unfortunately the method used then and even now that associates actual heart rates to maximum heart rates was not user friendly. The new Heart Theory of Exercise and Cardiofitness provides a more scientifically-accurate and easier to use method.

A Common Misconception is that a measured heart rate means a high heart rate, and when using so-called moderate exercise, it is not necessary to measure them. This is wrong. As I noted before, it can be more important to measure heart rates during low and moderate exercise than at high exercise. Exercise such as jogging or running entails moderately high heart rates. There will be little doubt that cardiofitness benefits are being obtained. But walking can produce either very good benefits or minimal benefits. The only way to assure benefits is to assure that a heart rate elevation of at least 30 to 40 beats per minute above low resting heart rate is being obtained.

I recently purchased a report from a prestigious medical school on how to exercise. Much of the report reflected today's conventional advice about exercise. But a glaring error was a sidebar stating that "Experts today say it is not useful to measure heart rates or to buy recording equipment to measure them." This is a sorry example of today's wrong advice about exercise. Because the exercise that protects health *develops* from maintained heart rate elevations. This is fundamental and casual. Without knowing our exercise heart rates we are exercising with the equivalent of random unmarked weights. We can have little idea about what we are accomplishing for either cardiofitness or health.

Try Measuring Your Heart Rate During the Day

An early step in developing your exercise program should be measuring your heart rate. Your heart is by far the most important organ in your body and you need to understand how it works. I hope that you already have obtained a measurement of your low resting heart rate as described in Chapter 4.

Please try taking your heart rate frequently for a day or two. You may be fascinated as I was to learn how it moves up during and after a meal, and then declines gradually over hours as the meal is digested. Start taking it when doing any kind of unusual physical effort to learn how your heart rate responds. A heart rate monitor can be very helpful. Try to get some idea of the highest heart rates you obtained during the day. It is that 2 hours per week or say 15-20 minutes each day of highest heart rates done regularly that mostly determines your cardiofitness.

If you are exercising to reduce weight, try taking your resting heart rate each hour after you finish exercising. Then compare these rates with those usual without exercise during the day. If you do any substantial exercise, you will view the calorie after-burn that is occurring after your exercise is done.

Heart Rates Vary During the Day

It is interesting to view how heart rates can vary during a typical day. Mike is a middle-age computer programmer that worked at a desk during the day. Thus without exercise he would qualify as a typical sedentary man. But he did do a real exercise session on this day, and had started doing this exercise intermittently. He has been fascinated about how his heart rate changes and uses his Polar Heart Rate Monitor frequently. He kindly provided me the charts that he developed during a typical day. Figure 13-1 shows heart rates in beats per minute taken during nine hours of the day followi his arrival at the workplace parking lot at 6:30 AM.

139

Figure 13-1

Heart Rates of a Middle Age Man During a Work Day

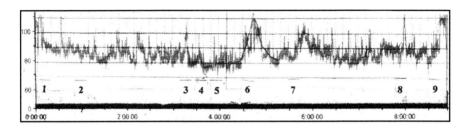

I have pasted some numbers at the bottom of the chart that identify things he did during this day. The plot shows heart rates in beats per minute at the left as hours of the workday advanced. The peak at (1) bottom left to a 110 heart rate reflected a long walk to and into the building. There was a drift downward during the morning from a usual 90 to about 80, which probably was due to the usual decline in heart rate as the morning meal was digested. A spike at (2) was a trip to the tea machine. Those at (3) and (4) were trips to the bathroom and for more tea. A lowest rate at (5) probably suggests the lowest resting heart rate obtained before lunch that averaged about 75. I do not have a low resting rate taken after getting up in the morning before breakfast but it probably was close to this value of 75.

At (6) he headed down 60 stairs to the cafeteria to buy a takeout lunch. You can see the increase in rate as he walked down stairs, the following short decline as he waited for the lunch, and the steep climb to a momentary rate above 120 as he ascended the 60 stairs again and ate his lunch. During the afternoon (7) he got up several times to walk around and talk to people. At (8) he went to the bathroom, and at (9) walked out of the building quite a ways to the parked car to go home.

Not shown in this chart, his heart rate followed a similar pattern of below about a 100 rate during dinner, followed by a decline to 80 as he rested afterward. It went into the 100-110 range when driving to an event after dinner and then down to a bit below 80 during subsequent reading.

During late evening his heart rate moved up to a near steady 140 beats per minute as he did 30 minutes on an exercise bicycle. It then dropped down rapidly before he went to bed. I understand that he had been doing this serious exercise only for a short time, and was doing it intermittently.

His general level of heart rate and probable low resting rate were somewhat higher than those of most people, but even with this bias his rate seldom went much above the 100 level during the day. Walking to and from the job provided a few minutes at about a 110 level, which represented a heart rate elevation above resting rate of 35.

Some Observations about These Heart Rates

How does knowledge of these heart rates help? The new Heart Theory views as important the highest exercise heart rates obtained during two hours of a week. This type of a record can identify the highest heart rates obtained during daily living. With exception of his exercise session, the highest usual rates obtained by Mike was about 110, and only about 30 minutes was spent with a heart rate above 100. I estimate that without the bicycle, his highest 2 hours per week would be at a heart rate of about 105. This is a heart rate elevation of 30 beats per minute above the likely low resting heart rate.

The Master Tables in Appendix one suggest that this 30 elevation for two hours a week would produce a CFR increase of about 6 from a usual base level of 90. This would forecast a probable CFR without exercise of 96. This is close to average for his age and quite typical for a person that does little planned aerobic exercise. We do not know his actual CFR.

The interesting question now is, What did his exercise session probably contribute? This exercise session produced a steady 140 average heart rate for 30 minutes. Four of these sessions per week would produce from the Master Tables at this 65 elevation in heart rate (140 exercise rate minus 75 low resting rate) an increase in CFR of about 19 or 19%. This exercise, done on 4 days each week, should provide after a year a 109 CFR and a very substantial health benefit vs. the 96 level estimated without this exercise. If this exercise is permanently maintained, it could lead to 4½ more years of healthy days of life and many more days that would be better.

It is interesting to reflect how the bicycle exercise could be the defining thing that will determine his cardiofitness. Two hours of this during a week would provide a stress on the cardiovascular system that was far higher than any other usual exercise he performed. If we think of the analogy of weightlifting, his bicycle exercise was the heaviest weight lifted, and is the key exercise that would produce cardiofitness.

The other physical activities he performed that were much lesser weights simply drop out of contention and do not matter much. Assume that he was awake for a usual 16 hours during the day. If we compute the calories of each activity during the day, the calories of the half hour on the bicycle would be far less than the calories burned during the other 15.5

hours he was awake. But these other calories that are by far the largest fraction of his total activity calories simply will not contribute much. Only the half hour at the higher level of 140 heart rate when he was on the exercise bicycle counts usefully to producing cardiofitness. This explains in another way why calories of physical activity do not relate usefully to the development of cardiofitness.

Is Continuous Heart Rate Monitoring Good?

Heart rate monitoring such as this may be a requirement for usefully valuing the effectiveness of exercise done in sports such as tennis or basketball or baseball. I mentioned that this could a valuable way to learn how cardio exercise develops in resistance training. It could be useful for valuing any other physical activity that involves intermittent expenditures of energy and varying levels of heart rate. This continuous monitoring requires a continuous record that can be printed out.

But monitoring requires equipment that is not inexpensive, and I found that getting a computer-associated monitoring device to work correctly to be a somewhat formidable task. A simple monitor that reads out heart rates should provide an adequate help to most people. The best heart rate monitors include a transmitter that is strapped to your chest that transmits values to a wristwatch type device.

But you can take your heart rate for 10 or 15 second periods easily yourself. Most aerobic exercises produce fairly consistent heart rates that can be easily measured in real time. Unless you have an occupation that produces appreciable energy demands, the cardiovascular benefit from today's usual lifestyle probably will be minimal. The only exercise of consequence will be the specific exercise that raises heart rates significantly for at least 2 hours per week such as what was done by Mike on his exercise bicycle.

Once you have a good idea of how a given exercise produces a heart rate, you will need to recheck measurements only occasionally. Exercise programs that use work stations, as for example in the Curves exercise outlets or in aerobic dancing, do provide for regular heart rate measurement. But this can be done manually. By recording the heart rates at each exercise station and averaging them you can obtain a useful value for your exercise heart rate elevation vs. low resting heart rate. Or you just can estimate your average heart rate from the measurements you made for 10 seconds. With a recognition of the heart rate target you wish to achieve for cardiofitness, you should just try to keep your heart rate close to this target during exercise.

CHAPTER 14.

STEP COUNTS AND CARDIOFITNESS

Step Counts Are Getting Increased Attention

The measuring of the number of steps taken each day via a pedometer has become popular recently. Some experts are excited about the possibility that these Step Counts can be a marker of the health value of exercise. I even see that a book has been written about this. A number of research papers have been published on how many steps different groups of people take each day. Some experts have suggested that 10,000 steps per day are needed for "good exercise."

You develop your Step Counts by wearing a pedometer on your waist. Values usually are recorded as full counts for a day, or for an average count done per day from counts taken on several different days. Most daily physical activity is done by moving about on foot. Step Counts thus provide a measure of the physical activity in a usual day. But pedometers, especially inexpensive ones, can be very inaccurate. You must confirm that one is producing correct and consistent values for distances walked before accepting its results.

Population Step Counts

A number of research studies have reported the average step counts of various populations. I have seen no analysis that identifies why these counts vary. Some values from these studies: Groups of US doctors averaged about 5,000/day. A group of 76 US men averaged 7,200/day and a related group of 133 women averaged 5,200/day. Some Japanese men averaged 10,000 on workdays and 7,100 on holidays. Some US men in a housing development averaged 5,300/day. A group of 57 diabetic men averaged 3,300/day.

A value of 4,000-6,000 seems typical of our US population of ages 30-60. But an Amish man was measured at 18,400 steps per day, and an Amish woman did 14,200. The Amish live a farming type of life similar to that lived by much of our population before about 1900. It seems likely that the populations that lived then produced not only much more physical activity but also produced such activity at higher intensities than are usual today.

Step Counts Can Be Helpful

Step Counts can provide a simple way for people to learn that they are physically inactive. It takes a usual 2000 steps to walk one mile. Fewer than about 4,000 to 5,000 Step Counts each day provides a warning that a person may not be doing enough exercise. Thus people that think they exercise enough can be shocked to learn that their say 3,500 daily steps represents solid evidence that their exercise is sadly lacking. Step Counts can useful when they stimulate an individual to initiate a useful program of exercise.

Aerobic and Anaerobic Step Counts

Step Counts will include both aerobic and anaerobic steps. Aerobic steps are those of walking or running that are developed for a some continuing duration. It takes about one minute of a continued exercise to elevate the heart rate sufficiently to produce useful cardiofitness. It takes about three minutes of continued exercise for heart rate to become fully elevated at a given intensity. Most steps taken around the home or work place are anaerobic steps taken for much shorter time periods than a full minute. These steps produce little if any contribution to exercise of the cardiovascular system.

The only steps that contribute usefully to cardiofitness and health are aerobic steps of moderate or vigorous walking or jogging or running. Please look at Table 2-3 and Figure 2-1 in Chapter 2 to view how risk of heart disease is reduced by various walking speeds and durations based on our largest epidemiology studies. Walking at speeds less than 1.5 miles per hour – and this will include anaerobic Step Counts – contributes little to reducing risk of heart disease. This is due to the fact that it requires at least a moderate walking pace continued for some time to increase the heart rate sufficiently to improve cardiofitness.

Anaerobic steps develop some small amounts of physical activity that can contribute to weight loss. More about this later. A person can develop a first 4,000 of mostly anaerobic Step Counts per day from walking about the house and workplace as part of daily living. These Step Counts usually produce little useful cardio or health benefit beyond that needed to keep sedentary people alive and well. Step Counts above about 4,000 per day suggest that useful aerobic walking for some distance probably is being achieved. Each added 2,000 Step Count above this 4,000 level usually identifies an added mile of potentially useful walking.

There is a Limit to the Aerobic Step Counts that are Useful

Two problems with Step Counts are first that they do not identify the intensity of exercise that is so vitally important to the development of cardiofitness. Second, only two hours per week of cardio exercise produces useful cardiofitness or health benefit. Thus high values of Step Counts usually will include large amounts of walking that are much beyond the two hours that is effective for improving health. This limit was shown in Chapter 2 and is more extensively verified in Appendix 3. The cardio system can absorb the benefits of only about 2 hours per week of cardio exercise..

2,000 Step Counts per day develops 14,000 per week or 7 miles of walking each week. If a person walks at a brisk 3.5 miles per hour, he or she would develop the needed 2 hours (7 miles divided by 3.5 mph) of walking from just 2,000 Step Counts per day. The cardiofitness and health value of these steps will depend on the average walking pace developed during this two hours of walking.

This identifies a new and surprising fact. Just 2,000 Step Counts each day done at a brisk walking pace of 3.5 miles per hour will develop close to the maximum usual benefit potential from walking at this pace. From Table 2-3 in Chapter 2, this maximum benefit from Step Counts and a 3.5 mile per hour pace of walking should produce a risk factor for heart disease of 0.56, or a reduction in risk of 44%. This maximum benefit for walking at 3.5 miles per hour translates into about a 9% improvement in cardiofitness. Because more than 2 hours per week will not produce more cardio benefit, more Step Counts that this 2,000 per day done at a given average intensity will produce no further reduction in risk of heart disease. This raises a serious question about value obtaining of such high values as 10,000 Step Counts per day.

The Research on Step Counts Verifies This

A most comprehensive-yet study published in Japan measured how the cardiofitness of 514 healthy persons that did little or no other exercise related to Step Counts.[38] Four study groups included both men and women of ages 30-49 and ages 50-69. The cardiofitness levels as VO2 Max of those having the lowest, median and highest daily Step Counts were measured for each group. Each group included results for 27 to 60 individuals.

The least active groups averaged about 4,000 Step Counts per day. The most active groups averaged about 10,000 Step Counts per day. Each of the more active groups thus developed about 6,000 more daily Step Counts than did the least active groups. Each of the high Step Count groups obtained a VO2 increase of about 9% and an improvement in CFR of 9 units compared with the low Step Count groups. This confirms that the high Step Count groups obtained close to my first suggested goal for improving cardiofitness of 10%.

At first glance these results appear very good. But the real question is, "Do Step Counts identify something different than the known effect of usual walking on cardiofitness?" The answer to this appears to be No. We have the excellent relationships between walking pace and duration on the risk of heart disease from our largest-yet studies in Table 2-3 of Chapter 2. It is of interest to compare these usual relationships for walking with results obtained from Step Counts.

The Research on Step Points Verifies
Previous Research Findings about Walking

We do not have the necessary information on how much or how fast the various individuals in the Japanese study walked. But the approximately 4,000 typical Step Counts of the low Step Count groups are consistent with those of inactive individuals that do little walking above the anaerobic walking needed for a usual lifestyle. The large advantage of the high Step Count groups could only have been a result of a large amounts of normal aerobic walking beyond that needed for usual lifestyle. Their approximately 6,000 additional Step Counts vs. those of the low Step Count groups required at a usual 2,000 Counts per mile about 21 miles each week of walking. Those that walk this large amount would probably have been walking quite briskly. At a brisk 3.5 miles per hour, this means that the active groups walked 6 hours more each week than did the inactive groups.

How does this benefit for 6 weekly hours of walking compare that for the two hours per week of brisk walking found previously to be effective for reducing the risk of heart disease? Table 2-3 in Chapter 2 showed from results of combined major studies that just 2 hours per week of brisk 3.5 miles per hour walking would produce a reduction in risk of heart disease of 43%. Each of the groups in the Japanese study developed about a 9% increase in VO2 or CFR that would reduce risk of heart disease by about 44%.

Thus the Japanese walkers obtained the same actual cardiofitness benefits and probable reduction in risk of heart disease from their 6 hours per week of added walking as would be expected from just 2 hours per week of usual brisk aerobic walking. Note that this Japanese research was not just one study. Results on four groups including both men and women of differing ages obtained essentially the same result. This provides a very close confirmation of the value of brisk walking previously developed in Table 2-3.

But this also confirms once again that more than two hours per week of walking produces no further cardiofitness benefit. The Japanese obtained the same likely reduction in risk of heart disease and cardio benefit from an average of six hours of walking each week as was obtained in major epidemiology studies for walking just two hours per week. This provides still another confirmation of the fact that only about two hours per week of aerobic exercise will be effective in reducing risk of heart disease and improving cardiofitness.

We thus have a scenario of a probable 2,000 aerobic steps producing the key benefit, and the additional 4,000 daily steps of the active group probably producing little cardio health value. This does not endorse a value for doing 10,000 or similar large amounts of Step Counts. Most of these high Step Counts appear to have produced little if any confirmed health benefit while consuming large amounts of exercise time. Doing just the 2 hours per week of brisk walking would have produced the same cardio and health benefits obtained from the time-consuming 6,000 additional daily Step Counts.

Step Counts Can Be Misleading

Step Counts can be useful in getting very inactive people to start doing more walking. Many studies show that Step Counts can reduce weight and cholesterol and improve other risk factors. But this research on Step Counts really provides only more data on the benefits of usual walking that accomplishes these same benefits. Considered in isolation and without the benefit of what we know about exercise, this research endorses Step Counts as good to do. Sufficient Step Counts as per the above study can produce close to the 10% improvement in cardiofitness that I cite is a first goal for improving health from exercise.

But just getting Step Counts can be an enormously inefficient method of exercise. Just 2,000 Step Counts or any other equivalent exercise done for two hours each week at the intensity of brisk walking each week produces the maximum improvement of the cardio system. Recall that the massive Step Counts of the mail carriers produced nearly the same reduction in risk of heart disease as did just 2,000 usual steps per day in other research on brisk walking.

Step Counts fail to quality as scientific for three reasons. They assign the same credit to near useless anaerobic steps as they do to steps of high-intensity productive aerobic walking. They assign a presumed value for steps for much longer than the two hours per week that is useful for improving the health of the cardiovascular system. They fail to teach the key value of higher walking pace in improving health risk.

It would seem more productive to target valuable exercise time to doing the exercise that best improves health. A more useful Step Count approach could be to develop a specific 2,000 Step Counts per day or an average 18 minutes each day of actual aerobic walking at a faster than usual walking pace. Time spent doing aerobic walking beyond this 2000 daily steps could be used for resistance exercise that improves other body muscles. Or, for those able, the walking could be replaced with other exercise that is more effective in improving health, as for example CARDIO 120.

Time spent doing Step Counts can help somewhat in weight reduction. But research shows that little reduction in weight develops from moderate walking without associated diet control. Otherwise, calories subtracted from diet tend to be "eaten up." Also and as noted previously, the calorie burn from walking is discouraging low unless it is done very briskly or fast.

Step Counts Can Be Fun

It can be interesting to see how many steps we take doing various activities. I wore a pedometer on a 12-day cruise once, and found that I walked an impressive total of 45 miles on the cruise. This was mostly due to walking to meals and events around the ship. It can be interesting to test how far we walk doing various types of physical activities.

In conclusion, Step Counts can be useful as a motivating tool that shows people how little they may be exercising. They might provide some people a basis for doing all of the exercise that will be acceptable to them. They could give older people that now do little exercise a first useful exercise goal. But it will be better for most healthy people to spend their exercise time doing the time-effective exercise programs described in this book. They will produce higher confirmed cardiofitness and improvements in health in a far more efficient time.

PART 5

EXERCISING TO A LONGER AND BETTER LIFE

CHAPTER 15

Answering the Many Questions

Our Physical Activity Has Been Dying

It is interesting to reflect how over my own lifetime our population physical activity has been declining. Before the 1960's, nearly every homeowner in our town had a lawn. We had those old push lawnmowers, the kind without any motor that got clogged up and was hard to push. Buying a power mower was thought of as absurd. These were for golf courses and commercial buildings. No one in the neighborhood had them. One would be ashamed to own one.

Yet a dozen years later everyone was making a racket with power mowers. The old push mowers were gathering rust. But the idea then that an ordinary homeowner would pay for a lawn service was outrageously extravagant. The first wimps to do this were regarded as lazy jerks.

Another dozen years later, nearly everybody in the neighborhood has a lawn service. Similarly, nearly every other physical task has been replaced with a power option. Power drills, power saws, power screwdrivers, power everything.

The kids that formerly walked to school a mile or even less now are driven there. Nearly every youngster that reached driving age has a car. Steadily, the BMI – that index of our weight – moved up. Just as steadily, the CFR or cardiofitness ratio of our population was moving down. And the health people were telling us more and more that we had to "exercise." And that we had to "lose weight."

No Single Exercise Program Is for Everybody

But as before, no canned program of exercise such as "Everyone should just walk a half hour or an hour everyday" can be appropriate for every man and woman of every age. Telling healthy young adults of age 20 or 30 to do only this seems absurd. These people should be doing much more vigorous exercise than usual walking. They should be getting their bodies into good physical and cardiofit shape for a physically active future life. They should be doing real heart-rate-monitored cardio aerobic exercise two hours each week and regular resistance exercise. They should be exercising sufficiently to produce a real improvement in the cardiofitness that can be most important of life-style actions that can improve their health.

As adults progress into older age – and I mean to ages of 70, 80 and even 90 – they should be doing good cardio exercise that is at least the equivalent of 4 mile per hour walking or better. If they started doing good exercise when younger, most of our older population should have little problem in doing this level of exercise into old age. Doing this will keep them out of walkers and wheelchairs for a decade.

Exercise recommendations should be targeted to produce a maximum health gain for our entire population. Until recently, recommendations for walking were targeted partly on the theory that the key group needing help was the 20% or so that were most unfit. More realistically, probably only 20% of our population is now exercising adequately. It is the remaining 80% that need to become more cardiofit.

Exercise Is for Life

Our life-style habits can be the #1 thing we can do that can reward us with a long, vigorous and disease-free life. Diet, exercise and no smoking rank at the top of these habits. But health habits must be maintained for life. Our risk of a heart attack or cancer can be dozens of times higher when we are older than when we are younger. It is of small benefit to avoid eating salt and excessive saturated fat during our 40's and then forget about doing this during later years.

Similarly, adequate cardio-oriented exercise must be done for life.

We need to think of our exercise as a regular and mandatory component of healthy living. I suggest following the many different kinds of exercise that can provide this benefit. Forget any idea that you can get your needed exercise from a lifestyle, as for example occasional gardening and bowling or even an hour everyday of slow walking.

Vigorous sports or marathons can produce high cardiofitness in your 20's and 30's, but will you keep this up every month in every future year? You need to think about things you will keep doing in your 70's, 80's and older. You can change exercises and their amounts and level as you become older. But you need to do meaningful exercise every week and every month of every year.

Exercise Is for Cardiofitness, Not Just for Weight

Much of the US population today is obese. People yo-yo in and out of diet programs to reduce weight. They also move on and off accompanying exercise programs for the same reason. There is an objective of losing some amount of weight. Once that objective is obtained, or the weight program is given up, the exercise stops. Exercise can be thought of as mostly something that helps people lose weight by burning calories. This is wrong.

Exercise usually can produce far larger health benefits by improving cardiofitness than by reducing weight. There has been much argument about this in recent years from some confusing research. There are exceptions. A 700-pound person has little alternative except to reduce weight. Reducing weight is #1 for the seriously obese because they probably cannot do the exercise needed to improve cardiofitness usefully until they slim down. But for the typical person that say is 50-100 pounds or less overweight, cardiofitness becomes the #1 action for improving health.

The Life Ahead computer model that should represent today's state-of-art technology from the most important published research provides useful answers about this for men or woman of any age. We can test from this model the health value of improving cardiofitness by 10% and 20%, which are the goals for exercise used in this book, and compare this with the health value of weight loss from the same exercise. The model forecasts that the gains in our future healthy days for reducing weight are only about 15% to 20% of the gains potential for improving our cardiofitness.

Exercise thus is not just something that is part of a weight reduction program. It is something that needs to be done all of the time and for a different reason. Exercise for cardiofitness combined with diet control can substantially help weight management. Higher cardiofitness also can help you burn more calories from a given time of exercise.

I have no intention here of demeaning the importance of weight loss. Large reductions in weight from serious obesity can produce major contributions to health. But diet is the BIG THING that reduces weight. Without diet control, exercise may not help weight management very much.

Exercising Safely

Exercise involves some risk. As intensity of exercise increases, this risk increases further. Although risks of exercise usually are tiny when compared to its benefits, everyone doing exercise should know that risks can be involved. They should reduce these risks as much as possible.

Joggers and runners and those doing other exercises do occasionally drop dead of coronary heart attacks. Twelve people died this way in Rhode Island between the years of 1975 to 1980. It was calculated that their risk of dying while running was 7 times higher than that of average people during the actual time they were running. Yet I computed that their absolute risk of death from coronary disease was only 1/20th of that of the average population there of their age. And the victims composed only 1 in 1760 of the individuals that had been running regularly. About half of the victims had pre-determinable coronary disease before they started running and had not visited or heeded their doctors.

James Fixx who wrote the top-selling Book of Running dropped dead of coronary disease. He also was found to have had almost completely clogged arteries related to a dismally high family history risk. He had not visited a doctor despite repeated advice to do so from associates that were concerned because of his other habits. I was particularly saddened by this because Jim had written such a favorable commentary on the cover of my earlier Random House book on exercise and cardiofitness.

A panel of the American Heart Association met recently to review research on heart attacks during physical activity. They found that people over 40 who died suddenly during exercise were mostly men with atherosclerosis in their coronary arteries that were unfit. They typically were sedentary but engaged in strenuous activity that they were not accustomed to do.

There are several things everybody that exercises should do.

1. Check your family history for risk of cardiovascular disease. Do you have a parent or grandparent that suffered? How about brothers or sisters?

2. Have your doctor look you over before you start any new or more intense exercise. Be sure to discuss your family history with the doctor if it is unfavorable, and to emphasis that you plan to exercise.

3. Move your exercise level up only very gradually. You can't get their faster than at the rather slow rate that your muscles will accept. Keep exercise at a given level for at least a week or two, or for a half dozen or more exercise sessions. Then move that exercise intensity up only gradually.

4. Listen carefully to your body at all times. If you feel anything different such as a slight pain and discomfort somewhere, or feel tired or a bit exhausted, stop immediately and rest a bit. Exercising for health is not a competition. There is no need to push yourself.

5. If you have not been able to exercise for a while, start up again slowly and carefully. It may take a month or two to get back to your previous shape.

6. There is an unverified but implied risk that moves up with higher exercise heart rates. This is a reason for those recommendations to exercise no higher than say 85% to 90% of maximum heart rate. Keep in mind that both the American Heart Association and the American College of Sports Medicine have endorsed use by healthy adults of exercise heart rates to 85%-90% of maximum heart rate. But these heart rates are not suitable for those that have not been exercising regularly for a few months.

    We should keep exercise at as modest an intensity as is necessary to improve cardiofitness. We usually do not want to develop heart rates moving from 100 to 140 back to average 120 because the implied risk at 140, even if tiny, is higher than the 120 rate. Those recommendations to exercise at levels of 50% to 90% of maximum heart rate are far too broad. These could include exercise that was too low for benefit and much higher than needed for those that have not been exercising vigorously.

7. Keep your exercise intensity from going suddenly high. This is particularly important in running. Jim Fixx died running up a hill. Moving up a hill or incline can increase your exercise intensity enormously. A monitored heart rate can teach you this. This risk can apply to walking up hills. If you start getting out of breath, think about this and stop for a bit.

Heart Rate Monitoring Is a MUST! The new Heart Theory of Exercise and Cardiofitness has reaffirmed the major importance of exercise heart rates. I have said this repeatedly. I see the failure to endorse heart rate monitoring as the single major mistake in much present advice about exercise. This lack of attention to exercise heart rates is an example of the steady regression away from good science about exercise during the past two decades by many so-called exercise experts.

Without a measured heart rate, our exercise is really a guess. I read ideas like "Exercise until you work up a sweat." I see this as nonsense. In hot humid climates you can be sweating before you even start your exercise. And in low humidity you can exercise more strenuously than you should and still not work up a sweat. Our health establishment is trying to teach exercise intensity without use of heart rates. The idea here seems to be that there are only two levels of exercise. One called moderate and the other vigorous. I wonder how many people can understand from this confusing advice how to exercise at either level.

One prominent and firmly opinionated exercise expert long ago told us that we did not need to measure heart rates. He advocated, "Just listen to your body. It will tell you when you get to the correct exercise level." I have listened intently, but sorry to say I never have heard anything useful.

I have highlighted an exercise heart rate of 120 beats per minute. This will produce useful gains in cardiofitness for nearly everyone. And it should be a safest usual heart rate than can develop and maintain useful cardiofitness. I told about my experience in getting to a very high CFR from exercising at or below this 120 exercise heart rate for many years. I believe that many others can take advantage of enjoying the fascinating dynamics of cardio feedback. Over a long time, this can result in steadily improving cardiofitness from exercise at a firmly monitored moderate heart rate. But if you have not exercised, please don't start by exercising even at that 120 heart rate. Start lower and work up slowly.

This monitoring of exercise intensity produces cardiofitness most efficiently. Keep in mind that the two hours per week of the most intense heart exercise you do produces over time the level of your cardiofitness. If you let the rate go up and down too much, the time that the rate is down may not count much in producing this cardiofitness.

What About Numbers of Sessions and Time of Sessions?

Research has verified that exercise in two segments at equal intensity for say 15 minutes is equivalent to one session at 30 minutes. This means you can divide your exercise time into convenient times. There probably is a limit here because it can take about three minutes for the heart to reach a plateau rate. Thus I would not suggest that a multiplicity of 5-minute segments would add the same way.

Research on resistance exercise has suggested that a day of rest between exercise sessions is desirable. Muscles need some time to regenerate after stress. I feel a bit better and exercise seems a bit easier after a day of rest between sessions.

This means that three aerobic exercise sessions at 40 minutes each on say Monday, Wednesday and Friday would produce the two hours per week needed. If four 30-minute sessions are used, then one would have to be done without that day of rest. But this is a very minor problem. Six 20-minute sessions on six days of the week would produce the two-hour total. I now exercise every day in the morning before breakfast for about 18 minutes. It has become such a part of my daily routine that I rarely think much about it. I still also exercise a bit more intensively by swimming during the months when our outdoor pool here is open.

Keep in mind that all times I quote for exercise are for those for aerobic exercise at target-exercise intensity. You have to modify this to include resistance exercise. Some exercise programs involve much time for preparation, warm-up, and cool down. There is undressing, shower and dressing. Times of these other tasks will not contribute much to cardiofitness.

How About Age? Doesn't This Make a Big Difference?

The simple answer to this is a firm NO. One of the key benefits of cardiofitness is that it conveys at least equal percentage reductions in risk of disease to the elderly as it does to younger people. And because actual levels of risk are far higher for the elderly, this means they can gain more absolute health benefit from exercise than can younger people.

It is true that younger people can develop higher heart rates than can those older. But most men and women of all ages can reach the 110-120 exercise heart rate that I emphasize as useful. Most younger people probably can develop the 140 level that I feel is a highest usually needed exercise rate for development of cardiofitness for health.

159

The physical condition of the body usually declines with age. The absolute level of cardiofitness as measured directly by VO2 Max usually declines about 35% as age moves from 20 to 80, and the potential level of athletic performance declines similarly. The CFR recognizes this usual change. Yet most of older people can keep their CFR well above the average of 100 for age, and a sizeable fraction can keep it well above 120 CFR with a good continued exercise program.

Cardiofitness and heart-rate-monitored exercise should be taught in school. All persons concerned with their health should be doing at least the Cardio 120 program as outlined in this book. Many should be doing more vigorous aerobic exercise than this plus an accompanying resistance exercise.

Those of 40's and 50's who want to start exercise but have not been doing it face a different problem. They need to start more carefully and only after consulting their doctor. Most at these ages probably should start exercise by walking, with the pace moved up only gradually But at these ages most should move up to good cardio, expect to become reasonably cardiofit, and carry this condition into much older years. Most men and women of this age should plan to develop better improvements in CFR than those potential from brisk walking.

And how about those in their 60's, 70's, 80's and 90's? As before, these are the ages that can be helped most by cardio exercise. Their health risks are higher than when they were younger. But they still can reduce this higher risk by up to several times by good cardiofitness. Most – and I mean those up to and beyond 90 – can do real aerobic exercise regularly. It is their choice whether they wish to just walk at a substantial pace or do more vigorous exercise. But they should know the potential benefit of either. Those at these ages especially need the periodic review of their doctor.

My next door neighbor now is a small and delightful woman named Mary. She walks at a somewhat incredible rate of speed. She exercises nearly everyday on the treadmill. She moves the incline up to as high as it will go at the 15% grade and walks on it at at above 3.5 miles per hour. People passing by are awed to see her walking so fast up what appears to be a very steep hill and leaning backwards. I don't know her CFR but it must be extremely high. Mary was 87 years old when I first saw her doing this.

Is That Two-Hour Time for Aerobic Exercise Accurate?

The answer here is that it is approximate. A close look at the data we have suggests that this time could be between 1.7 and 2.3 hours. It probably will vary by intensity of exercise, but I could not find enough data to verify this. For example, the maximum exercise time at stress that is useful in improving muscle in resistance exercise appears to be much less than this two hours each week and may be closer to only 30 minutes each week. It is possible that there may be a daily as well as a weekly limit to the rate at which cardiofitness can improve. Thus I would not suggest a single two-hour session each week, or even two one-hour sessions.

Our database is from individuals that mostly exercised several times each week. The first hour per week of exercise may produce 60% of the potential benefit of longer exercise. As before, an hour and a half per week may produce 86% of the maximum potential benefit. Thus if you exercise 90 minutes each week, you may obtain most of the benefit for the full two hours. You might recapture the remaining benefit from some aerobically-oriented resistance exercise.

A time suggested in various exercise programs today is 20 minutes of cardio on three days of the week. This totals only one hour and gives 60% of potential aerobic benefits. If exercise heart rate is about 120 beats per minute and your resting heart rate is 70 or higher, this time of exercise usually is not sufficient for obtaining a good cardiofitness in one year. If you can exercise comfortably and safely at an exercise heart rate of 140 beats per minute, you can achieve reasonably good cardio benefits from one hour per week at this rate. See again Table 5-1 in Chapter 5 for the improvement in CFR you should obtain from various exercise heart rates by just one hour of exercise per week. Or use the Master Tables in Appendix 1 for cardiofitness development at different exercise heart rates.

I Had a Heart Attack but I'm Completely Recovered. Should I Do the Same Exercise?

My position is that anyone that suffers a cardiovascular related disease or any other disease should be guided first by the advice of a doctor. All of the re-search I have seen – and there is a lot of it – says that exercise reduces the risk of future disease similarly for those that have and for those that have not suf-fered a cardio disease. But exercise involves increased risks for those that have suffered this disease, and exercise by those having had it usually should be done in a medically monitored facility until the doctor advises otherwise.

I Am Diabetic. Can Exercise Help?

Chapter 7 showed that exercise, and especially that producing cardiofitness, provided substantial protection against diabetes. Other research shows that exercise also can reduce blood glucose and is a part of the therapy for diabetes usually suggested by doctors. Exercise done before a meal may have little benefit in reducing glucose level. Research suggests that exercise after a meal may be best for this purpose. If you are diabetic, you will have to try this out yourself, but be sure to get the doctor's advice. One suggestion is to carry around a glucose- rich snack in the event your blood glucose goes too low during exercise.

I have arthritis in my legs I cannot walk fast.

The simple answer here is swimming. Swimming can exercise other body muscles that can keep exercise heart rate elevated usefully. If you cannot swim or have no place to do it, an exercise professional might be able to help you.

I cite the following results of some smaller studies that showed various potential benefits of exercise. Studies like these usually do not provide us a useful measure of what kind or amount of exercise was involved. But most of them show results for what probably was rather modest differences in cardiofitness.

Exercise can Lower Stress:

Exercise can take your mind off of troubling problems and give you a time-out from them. It may break down the hormones and other chemicals that build up during periods of intense stress. The electrical activity of tense muscles decreases measurably after a bout of exercise.

Exercise Can Improve Your Mood

Studies indicate that exercise can be as effective as some antidepressants in treating mild depression. Moderately depressed persons who engage in aerobic exercise often experience a mood change after two to three weeks of exercise. This may be due to changes in brain nutrition such as an increase in endorphins, and a decrease in cortisol and other stress hormones.

Exercise Can Be Sexercise!

At least one study found that exercise produces better sex. Men that exercised were five times as likely to achieve normal sexual function as were those that did not exercise.

Lack of Exercise Leads to ED. A study in the Journal of Urology in 2006 of 22,000 health professionals found that regular physical activity of any type reduced the risk of erectile dysfunction.

Exercise Can Reduce Insomnia

A moderate workout before bedtime can help some people get a full night's sleep. This may be a due to a reduction in stress hormones and anxiety that can disturb sleep.

Exercise Can Reduce Depression

Dr. James Blumenthal of Duke University reported that regular exercise could help eliminate depression as effectively as anti-depression medicines.

Exercise Can Improve Self-Image

Improving cardiofitness by cardio exercise or resistance exercise can develop self-confidence and self-esteem. It provides a sense of control over the body. Being able to walk easily and briskly at ages 80 and 90 can keep your self-image satisfyingly high when viewing that most of your peers are walking slowly with canes and walkers.

Exercise Can Improve Mental Performance

Researchers at the Salk Institute for Biological Studies in San Diego have reported that there is growing evidence that regular and consistent exercise can improve cognitive performance in both young healthy individuals and in older individuals.

Exercise Can Reduce Risk of Upper Respiratory Infections

A study found that a good walking program reduced the risk of infections roughly in half. Immune cells can remain elevated for three hours after a good walking session.

Some Exercises That Are Not Sufficient

There are misconceptions about what exercise is and what it means to health. My friend George recently told me firmly that he had DONE his exercise. He had worked on a factory floor for 20 years doing hard physical labor. "You should have seen the exercise we did then!" he said. The implication was that he had done it then, and that was enough for life.

It could have been pointless to suggest to opinionated George that the kind of factory physical activity he probably did would not improve cardiofitness very much. And that any advantage that he obtained then probably was gone six months after he had retired eight years ago. He was now doing zero useful exercise.

A substantial part of our population view exercise as things they do now that are physical and tiring. Yet a monitored heart rate such as that for Mike in Chapter 13 probably will show that most things they do probably will not move their heart rates up beyond 100 beats per minute for more than a few minutes a day. Some exercise experts tell about dozens of things they called exercise that can help us such as gardening, housework, golf, billiards or pool, painting and even fishing. This just continues the misconception about what is really useful cardio exercise.

It has been pointed out that any kind of exercise can help those that are in extremely poor shape. For example, a walk across the room can be a major exercise for someone long bed ridden. People formerly ill may get major benefit from even the slowest walking. This book is oriented to help otherwise normal healthy people do the exercise that can make a real improvement in their long range health.

Cardiofitness requires exercise affecting the entire cardiovascular system of heart, arteries, capillaries and veins that provides oxygen to the cells of our body. Without this system functioning, we will stay alive only a very few minutes. It delivers not only oxygen but an enormous population of nutrients, vitamins, minerals and other bio-chemicals that fuel all functions of the body.

Exercise of this cardiovascular system is accomplished only by increased blood flow in and throughout this entire body. This requires significantly higher than usual heart rates maintained for significant times up to a total of two hours each week. Playing pool or doing some usual gardening each week simply is not going to accomplish this. There is a major need for people to know their cardiofitness. This and only this can tell them where they are on a health related scale of major importance to future life.

The providing of a widely available accepted simple test for cardiofitness that measures people's CFR – and a widespread understanding and acceptance of this CFR – could be the most important single public health action that this country and other developed countries could take.

Such a test – and only a simple test that is both easy to take and provides a direct single understandable number result such as the CFR – could finally wake up people to the importance of their cardiofitness. This could start a real revolution of cardiofitness.

In contrast, a technically oriented expensive cardiofitness test requiring medical oversight as a doctor's prescription and/or requires charts to develop researcher type values and risks would contribute relatively little to our population health.

It Is Aerobic Exercise That Comes First

A vast amount of talk about exercise today confuses what is important with what is vastly less important. We hear about exercises for flexibility, for upper-body or muscular strength, for changing body composition, for selectively reducing fat, for conditioning.

Kenneth Cooper said back in 1968 in his classic book Aerobics: "I'll state my position early. The best exercises are running, cycling, walking, stationary running, handball, basketball, and squash in just about that order. Isometrics, weight lifting and calisthenics although good as far as they go, do not even make the list." Many of today's so-called health experts need to go back and read his pioneering book. They still have not caught up to where he was 40 years ago.

Our focus today has shifted to a broader population from youth to beyond 90. Thus the basketball, squash and handball he discussed may not be appropriate for all. But the value of aerobic exercise has been reconfirmed overwhelmingly. This is the research that can substantially improve health. Resistance exercise can help further. But aerobic exercise remains as primary for future health.

The Exercises That Can Improve Cardiofitness

Practical exercises can produce the steady elevated heart rates needed to improve cardiofitness. These include walking, jogging, running, cycling, swimming and other water exercise. We also have the treadmill and exercise bicycle and aerobic dancing. We also have the many other exercise machines that either individually or sequentially in circuit-type training can help produce excellent aerobic exercise.

Walking

Walking must be the #1 of all exercises for health and cardiofitness. Most of those that are not reasonably cardiofit should start exercise by walking. The really BIG THING about walking is the importance of pace. Two hours each week at any pace is enough. Keep in mind that cardiofitness improves slowly. You cannot improve it faster than about 1% per week. Thus it is just as effective and much safer to start walking just a bit faster than usual for two weeks or full month. Then continue to increase exercise just modestly from time to time.

Walking as I said before can cost nothing in fees, can be done any time of the day, and often can be done near your home without having to drive somewhere. After a move that took me away from a fine indoor swimming pool, I started walking a fast mile and a half each morning before breakfast. This accomplished the needed two hours of exercise each week in about 18 minutes per day. It wakes me up and gives me a lift. And my low resting heart rate has stayed in the low 50's indicating my cardiofitness was being maintained at least approximately.

Look again at that Table 2-3 and Figure 2-1 in Chapter 2 that shows from very large studies how risk of heart attack declines with walking pace. Just walking without knowing your pace or heart rate may be wasting a lot of time. Once you know how your heart rate responds to exercise, you will need to recheck heart rates only occasionally. The values quoted for walking pace are for people of average height. Tall people will need to walk a bit faster and short people can walk somewhat slower than these averages for a similar benefit.

How Do You Measure Walking Distance and Pace

This can be a problem. Over the years I have used a half dozen pedometers. Most were very inaccurate. The last one I tried was more expensive than usual at about $25, and it did work better than others. But I still had to find the right place to wear it to get consistent readings. Test it for two to three days by walking the same distance to be sure it gives consistent results. You may have to try wearing it at different locations around your waist. If it does not give consistent readings for a given distance, it could be worthless.

You can lay out a measured distance and test how many steps this takes. With a little mathematics you can translate number of steps to a 5280-foot mile or to a kilometer if this is what you measure. Another way is to drive a half or full mile and note your terminal point. Then walk the same distance to get your pace. But for accuracy you have to watch the tenth-mile speedometer indicator closely to be sure it ends up in the same exact position as at start.

Many and perhaps most cities in the Midwest and West were designed in one mile grids, with major thoroughfares at mile positions and secondary thoroughfares at half-mile positions. Country roads are commonly set at such intervals. Check this out on your car speedometer.

Walking on the street or even crossing streets can be dangerous. It hardly is productive to be hit by a car when trying to improve your health. It is better to find a place to walk that is relatively free of vehicular traffic. And walking or doing any exercise on the street or road requires inhaling unwanted pollution. Many people today do their early morning walks in malls or parks.

Some Walking Tips

Stand tall. Keep your shoulders back, and tuck your abs to avoid arching your lower back. Increase your walking pace first by taking quicker steps. It takes more energy to move to longer steps, but you may need both quicker and longer steps to get your heart rate up. Usual walking trains only the legs. You can flex your hands during your walk to improve their flexibility. Try exercising your arms in different ways to obtain a little more muscle and flexibility.

Bend your arms up to a 90-degree angle. Keep your elbow fixed. Your hands should come only to the front of your body. Faster movement of arms may help increase pace and increase exercise intensity. Push off with your back foot for power. Use quality walking shoes and keep them in good shape.

Should you use weights when walking? This is controversial and many experts say no. But you can swing your arms when walking to gain some exercise intensity.

Is All Walking Aerobic Exercise?

Most walking qualifies technically. But realistically I view only that that develops at least a 30 beat per minute elevation in heart rate above low resting heart rate as usefully aerobic. Walking at speeds approaching 5 miles per hour can produce heart rate elevations of 50-60 beats per minute that in turn can produce excellent aerobic exercise and a quite healthful increase of 20% in cardiofitness. Speed walkers can go even faster. But being able to maintain such a walking pace also requires very good cardiofitness. Most people may find other kinds of cardio exercise more acceptable than very fast level ground walking.

Much about walking is now on the internet. For example check www. walking.org and www.thewalkingsite.com and others. Walking at any pace still does not accomplish the objectives of better overall physical fitness such as upper body strength, general body fitness or flexibility. This requires resistance exercise.

Walking with Poles

Walking with poles, or so-called Nordic walking, can improve the cardiofitness effectiveness of walking. Two published studies found that groups that walked with poles acquired at similar perceived levels of exertion more than a 20% higher improvement in their VO2 Max and CFR than did similar groups that walked without poles. Cooper Institute researchers found that walking with poles burned 40% more calories and produced higher exercise heart rates than those that walked normally. Walking with poles produced better upper-body exercise, less stress on knees and lower impact on the body.

I have never done this, but the research results regarding it are impressive. A variety of walking poles are advertised on the internet by different vendors, so many people now must be doing this.

Jogging

Jogging really is running, but running at a somewhat slow pace. If you keep walking fast, you may move into jogging automatically at a pace of about 5 miles per hour. This happens because at this crossover pace it actually can require a bit fewer calories of energy to jog than to walk. Jogging can include pace levels of 5-6 miles per hour before moving into full and still faster running.

Your feet do not leave the ground when walking. Jogging raises your foot off the ground at each step. Although jogging usually will produce higher heart rates than fast walking, speed walking at up to and past 6 miles per hour that forces you to keep your feet from leaving the ground can actually consume more energy and produce higher heart rates than will jogging at the same pace.

Jogging has a main benefit of further elevating the heart rate beyond that usual from walking. You cannot jog without usefully increasing your heart rate elevation, and jogging ensures that you will obtain cardiovascular benefit. But this comes at some cost. As you move into running from walking, the rate of injury from falls or muscle problems increases several-fold There is a more of shock and stress to the body as each step contacts the pavement. Some fitness experts are unenthused about jogging for this reason.

But as with walking, jogging does not require extra costs of club membership, and it can be done around the home at times most convenient. Done sufficiently for two hours per week, it essentially ensures that good cardiovascular improvement will be obtained. And this improvement can add several healthy years of life and is a vastly greater health benefit than the offsetting problem of what usually is a fairly modest and usually repairable injury. I did some jogging for many years as a supplement to my swimming, and fell twice. I was in some pain for a while, but the pain was soon gone.

A message here is just be careful if you jog or run. You do not have to fall. This usually happens from being inattentive. I fell both times from what obviously was inattention. I also damaged my knee from another fall that put me on crutches for almost a half year. Ironically this more serious fall occurred when putting up some outside Christmas lights. I was still able to continue my regular swimming when on the crutches.

An interesting use of jogging is doing it in combination with walking. For example, you walk 50 paces and jog 10 paces. Then walk 50 paces and jog 20 paces. Or go 50-50. You automatically will be walking very fast because the walking will tend to be on the verge of jogging. I did this for some years and found I liked it. It substantially reduced the stress from jogging and kept my heart rate up where I wanted it. Even the use of only 10 paces of jogging per 50 paces of walking helped in keeping my walking pace and heart rate up.

Running

This may be the #1 of all exercises that contribute to cardiofitness. Yes, it does contribute several times more falls and injuries than does walking. But any overall health debit for this must be trivial compared with the major benefits.

Running may be the best of all usual exercises that can reduce weight. Runners say that they obtain intense exhilaration and euphoria well into and after a run. This comes from a beta endorphin release triggered by the neurons in the nervous system that creates a feeling of extreme happiness and exhilaration. Runners claim to achieve more energy in daily life. And it helps bring appetite, exercise and food into balance. Because running makes the body function better, it improves sleeping, eating and relaxation.

Running can produce an exercise heart rate of 150 or higher for those of middle age or younger. This heart rate maintained over a time in years can develop very high fitness from 2 hours per week. Running just one hour each week can develop quite good cardiofitness. You don't have to run the marathon or hundreds of miles.

It simply makes no sense to run along narrow roads or on the interstate highways breathing in masses of vehicle fumes. Recent research showed that diesel fuel exhaust includes microscopic soot particles that were especially risky for people with heart disease and increase risk for those who otherwise are healthy. Runners can breathe in much more polluted air than walkers do.

Running can be a top exercise for the younger. But as people move into and beyond middle age, it should be done with increasing caution. Some can run comfortably into very advanced age. But running may not be a best exercise for most people much beyond age 60.

I personally never was a runner. A problem for runners is where to run to avoid contact with cars. Runners tend to go much longer distances than do those that walk. As with walking, jogging and running produce leg muscle but do not contribute much to overall body physical fitness or flexibility. There are alternatives to outside or track running that may produce similar cardiofitness benefits with lesser problems and risks, and that also can contribute similarly to cardiofitness. Again, a vast amount of information about running is on the internet and in magazines and books.

Lap Swimming

This has been my favorite exercise. It usually requires an indoor or heated pool for continuous year-round exercise. Swimming avoids the danger of outside exercise from pollution and motor vehicles It does not jar the body as does running. It involves fewer injuries.

I mentioned earlier that swimmers obtained much lower values of C reactive protein, or CRP, than did runners or those doing other sports.

This may result in less of the inflammation that can increase risk of heart disease. Swimming can develop a continued elevated heart rate that with practice can produce either moderate, intermediate or highest levels of cardiofitness.

A first problem for lap swimming is that you must be able to swim. I was a good swimmer and even did some life guarding in my youth. But I found that when trying it again during middle age, I no longer could swim more than one 25-yard pool lap without resting. It took several sessions – and it was learning again how to breathe properly – before I could make it much past that first lap without a rest. You just have to be patient and keep trying.

But eventually I did become comfortable doing multiple laps and I worked up to doing regular sessions of the 72 laps needed in the 25-yard pool to complete the mile in around 40-45 minutes. This is far longer than the time needed by the athletes to do this, but it kept my heart rate at a near steady 120 beats per minute. The result was exhilarating and a good shower afterward left me feeling great. I did this three times a week for nearly thirty years before slowing down somewhat. With a father that dropped dead of cardiovascular disease at age 45 I probably would not be here today if I had not done this regular swimming.

A problem in lap swimming is measuring your heart rate. My pool had a fine large clock with second hand that I could see and use. The experts recommend use of swimming goggles, but using them complicated seeing the clock. You can obtain equipment (see the internet) that measure heart rates in water. I strongly urge that if you do serious lap swimming, you arrange some method for solving this problem. You can stop and take a heart rate occasionally if you have a suitable waterproof watch, but there is the problem of being to able read it when your eyes are wet or in goggles.

Swimming one 25-yard pool length per minute probably will elevate your heart usefully. Three pool lengths in two minutes should produce very good aerobic exercise. And 2 lengths per minute puts you in the athletic range which should produce excellent conditioning for younger and middle-aged persons.

Swimming exercises the arms and upper body, improves flexibility and reduces stress, but it may not exercise the legs or other body muscles very much. I do both freestyle and breaststroke alternately to get better thigh exercise. But I supplement this with about a half-hour per week of jogging or walk–jog combinations to get some better leg exercise. Even with this I was a bit dizzy when getting up from working near the floor. Brief sessions of 15 or 20 full knee bends a few times each week solved that problem.

Water's buoyancy makes it easy on joints and is particularly useful for those with joint problems such as arthritis. Swimming with a kickboard is especially good for strengthening the legs, but it's very demanding. The theory that swimming after a meal can produce stomach cramps appears to be largely disproved. But swimming after eating can hinder digestion. I found swimming after a meal to be uncomfortable.

Water Exercise

Many exercise programs today involve walking or exercising in the water. Water aerobics can produce excellent conditioning. Exercising in the water can produce higher heart rate elevations than doing the same thing out of the water, and lessen the problem of injury. It also keeps you way from cars and their emissions.

This is an area in which an instructor may be needed. The exercise can be done in group classes. Occasional classes may not make you very fit. And another problem with water exercise is that of measuring your heart rate when in the water. I feel that instructors of water exercise should occasionally help participants measure the heart rates, but I've not seen anyone do this.

Cycling

This refers to riding an actual bicycle on the street, road, or track. Riding a bicycle on a clear track can provide a monitored increase in heart rate and excellent cardio exercise. But finding a suitable track may be difficult. My opinion is that street bicycling is rarely useful for improved cardiofitness.

The problem is that you really must cycle away from the cars and trucks to improve your heart rate usefully. It can be impossible to develop cardiofitness by cycling in the streets of a usual town. You cannot pedal at a sustained pace because you need to stop for traffic at every cross street. Cycling on a road or highway is dangerous. And it can be impractical to measure a heart rate unless you wear a fairly expensive monitor with a chest transmitter.

Many years ago my wife and I decided we needed to exercise more and acquired two bicycles. We set off on the town streets. A car cut her off after about ten minutes and she was finished. She would never ride her bike again. I tried riding my bike a few more times but gave it up. It just did not work. There just were too many cars.

The Netherlands is the place where bicycles can be used effectively. Many streets have accompanying bicycle paths and those Dutch men and women really ride their bikes fast. The real danger there is to a pedestrian that gets in their way. But the US is not designed for bicycles. It is best to ride a stationary exercise bicycle here if you do not have a suitable track..

The Treadmill

This must be the #1 of all machines for exercising. It takes you off the street and away the cars and pollution. You can walk, jog or run on it. You can be injured, but the risk is lower than when running on the street. It permits you to walk and still achieve almost any desired heart rate by adjusting the incline. Thus your bones can avoid the jarring of jogging or running while you still achieve high levels of conditioning.

The better treadmills include devices for directly monitoring your heart rate. These can be very helpful. Treadmills have timers for monitoring your time, and indicators of your miles traveled. Some treadmills have attachments that can help exercise your arms. I had such a treadmill and found the arm exercise to be useful.

A good quality treadmill will monitor your walking pace. You also can adjust the incline at a given walking speed to develop a desired exercise heart rate and see this displayed directly on the monitor. Maintaining a desired exercise heart rate when doing normal street walking usually requires stopping and taking a heart rate by counting beats.

Treadmills are found in essentially every exercise facility. But you can buy your own and do your exercise without paying fees or having to drive somewhere. You can watch television or even read when doing your exercise. I strongly recommend that you get a good one that can set an accurate incline and that can measure heart rate accurately. Also pay attention to how much noise it makes. One I bought made so much noise that it was impossible to listen to the TV when it was in operation. A treadmill can sound a lot louder in your house than it does in the store.

You can program your exercise better with a treadmill. For example you can set your heart rate target up just marginally each week to assure you are not moving up too fast. Unless you are very cardiofit, you probably can achieve any heart rate you desire from walking at some level of incline.

The big problem with a treadmill – and this is true for any exercise machine – is that it can be so boring. Twenty minutes walking outside viewing the countryside and what is happening can pass by pleasantly. But twenty minutes on the treadmill looking at a wall can seem like forever. I strongly recommend watching the TV or reading or trying to do something else when exercising. Boredom can be a #1 reason why people stop exercising.

A few years ago my wife and I visited a Life Care facility where a friend and many other seniors were spending their final years. We were shown a large room filled with dozens of treadmills, bicycles and other exercise machines. Our friend told us that because their rooms were rather small, they could keep and use their exercise machines in that room to save space. I asked an obvious question: "How many people use these machines regularly?" The answer was: "Hardly anyone!"

This was sad. These were the people that needed exercise more than ever before in their lives. Many were moving from good walking to pushing walkers and using canes and wheelchairs. Using their machines could have delayed for years this sorry decline and added many more healthy days to their lives. But exercising in that large room must have been both lonely and incredibly boring. There had to be a better way for people to do their needed exercise.

The Exercise Bicycle

Much of what was said above for the treadmill applies to the exercise bicycle. This bicycle is stationary, and the user pedals at a selected speed and against an adjustable resistance load. By adjusting speed and load, a user can achieve and maintain a wide range of steady monitored exercise heart rates. Exercise bicycles come in a wide range of prices and sophistication, and some can measure heart rates and produce much information about cardiofitness. But the exercise bicycle really trains only the leg muscles and trains them in a specific way.

The exercise bicycle eliminates the hazards of being on the road, and does not put stress on the joints and bones as does running. It can take up less house space than does a treadmill. But for some reason I always preferred the treadmill. I understand that the public also much prefers treadmills. The exercise bicycle requires a focused leg movement that is not as familiar as walking on the treadmill. I found riding the exercise bicycle to be even more boring than the treadmill.

Aerobic Dancing

This was originated by Jacki Sorenson in 1968 and I long have felt it to be one of the greatest of all exercise programs. I was impressed by seeing Jacki and her demonstration group of incredibly fit women in the early 1980's. My wife participated for quite a few years and danced in some of Jacki's large demonstration programs. A typical aerobic dancing session involves 20-30 minutes of heart-rate-monitored exercise done to music, with much warm-up and cool-down time that can involve various stretching exercises.

It is claimed that 24 million women have participated in aerobic dancing programs. A typical program entails 3 sessions per week for 10 weeks, and 4 of these programs per year can provide near continuous year around exercise. The dances can be performed at home to videos. But most find exercising in classes to familiar music to be more fun than doing exercises on their own.

I think it is unfortunate that so very few men participate in this activity. Jacki's program includes sessions of three different exercise intensities. (See more on www.Jackis.com.) There are many other aerobic dancing programs offered nationwide by other sponsoring groups.

Many participants in these programs may do them more for weight management than for cardiofitness. With accompanying diet control the program can contribute effectively to reducing weight. But research has verified that aerobic dancing also can produce quite useful improvement in cardiofitness. One study showed an average gain in cardiofitness of 12 in CFR after 14 weeks of aerobic exercise. This exceeds my suggested first goal of 10 in CFR.

This aerobic dancing maintained for life at three sessions per week at a needed level of exercise could extend healthy life by nearly 4 years. An actual improvement will depend importantly on average time of exercise, exercise heart rate elevations during usual exercise and number of sessions done per week. The Cardiofitness Points method can provide a way to view likely cardio benefits from aerobic dancing.

A common suggestion in aerobic dancing is to exercise at 60% of maximum heart rate. As before, this 40-year-old "percentage of maximum heart rate" method using the usual formula is not a useful basis for monitoring heart rate. It is of use only for people younger than age 60. Values of 50% to 60% of maximum heart can absurdly specify zero exercise for those who are older because resting heart rates can absurdly be in this 50-60% range.

A more accurate and much easier method is to develop exercise heart rates of at least 110 to 120 beats per minute, as in CARDIO 120. This moderate level should be both useful and safe for medically approved persons of all ages that are conditioned for exercise. These heart rates are commonly developed in aerobic dancing. See Appendix 1 for the Master Tables that show how your cardiofitness will improve for various heart rate elevations maintained for different amounts of time per week. Then review using these tables how your heart rate elevations and time during aerobic dancing probably will develop cardiofitness.

The much lower heart rates obtained during warm up and cool down probably will not help much in increasing cardiofitness. If you exercise at elevated heart rates only 20 minutes per session, you probably will not obtain the two hours of exercise needed for desirable cardiofitness in three dances per week. You will need to do some other exercise as for example some aerobic dancing at home to obtain my suggested goals.

Sports

Young people who are regularly active in sports such as basketball or handball will generate the heart rate elevations sufficient to improve cardiofitness. But for non-athletes, most sports may contribute only modestly to health. As example, football develops short bursts of energy for perhaps 6-10 seconds per play followed by far longer times of standing and walking to new positions. This will not make you cardiofit.

There is an illusion that those that participate in sports must be quite fit. More accurately, tennis and most other sports done by those who are middle age can involve a lot of standing and walking about and may not improve cardiofitness usefully. Another problem is that some sports can be seasonal. Good aerobic exercise should be done continuously throughout the year.

Some of those tables of physical activity calories we find for different sports appear to have been developed from observing young athletes. As before, many calorie values in books and on the internet are the misleading Total Calorie values rather than the more meaningful Net Calories. A study I did some years ago suggested that average calories developed from sports were about one-third as effective in reducing risk of heart disease as were calories of steady aerobic exercise.

Because exercise heart rates fluctuate so much during sports activity, the only way that their contribution to cardiofitness can be measured is by using a continuous heart rate monitor. But I have not seen study results of this. Either an average heart rate taken during sports activity or an estimate of the highest rates often achieved can be used together with the Master Tables to produce such an estimate. The actual cardiofitness levels of sports participants can be measured by the methods outlined in Appendix 2.

Sports that should improve cardiofitness substantially are soccer and ice hockey. Participants move around nearly continuously at very vigorous levels in these sports. A study by Dr. Peter Krustrup, head of Copenhagen University's department of exercise and sport sciences, found that young soccer players appeared to gain better exercise test results than did runners. The soccer players reached exercise intensities of 90% of maximum heart rate, which were higher than those developed by the runners.

Sports are mostly played by those young. Because most of those that play sports discontinue this activity as they progress in age, sports rarely will compose a lifetime scenario for cardio exercise. The cardiofitness from sports probably will be mostly gone a half-year after the activity is stopped. Thus most of those that have felt comfortable with their fitness from sports need to consider another cardio type activity for their older age.

Exercise Machines

There is an enormous number of exercise machines today. Some claim to make you fit in 5 minutes per day or to help you lose 5 pounds per week. This is complete nonsense. Machines do not do any exercise for you. The only exercise that counts is what you do. Muscles will improve at their own pace, which cannot be increased by more exercise. Disregard those testimonials of what machines did for someone. And disregard any claims that a machine can selectively remove fat from one part of your body. Research does not support this.

Most machines can be divided into two categories. Those that help produce aerobic exercise, as do treadmills, bicycles, stepping and rowing machines, and those designed for resistance exercise. Some are designed for both types of exercise.

A potential benefit of specialized exercise machines is that they can be designed to improve more muscles than those improved by the aerobic exercise of treadmills and bicycles. As before, an optimum development of overall physical fitness would require the exercise of as many needed muscles as possible while at the same time producing continuous monitored cardio exercise. This probably will require some compromise in effectiveness of the individual exercises.

Circuit Training and Interval Exercise

This involves training at a series of exercise stations that are designed to both keep heart rate up and train as many other body muscles as possible. The earliest programs of exercise such as some started before 1970 did involve such circuit training. Some gym programs attempt to achieve this objective. The new Heart Theory of cardiofitness identifies some sharper and important objectives for such programs.

A first objective must be a practical number of weekly sessions that can develop and maintain a steady cardio heart rate elevation for two hours per week. A second objective will be to include exercise within this circuit of other parts of the body that can provide a broader range of flexibility and strength. The challenge is to include added useful exercise that holds overall exercise time to a minimum beyond this two hours

The Curves Exercise Program Provides Interval Exercise

The Curves program for women that started in 1992 aims to provide both aerobic and resistance exercise simultaneously and can accomplish useful benefit from both in a time of about two hours each week. They now claim 10,000 locations in 44 countries serving 4 million women and proclaim themselves the largest exercise franchise in the world.

Curves uses about a dozen exercise stations that are separated by platforms. The machines used for resistance training stress the major muscle groups in the body, some by both pulling and pushing. The women sit in a circle and are able to converse. Music plays and there are voice prompts every 30 seconds to change exercise stations. The participant spends 30 seconds on a resistance machine and then moves to another 30 second time interval, usually involving aerobic exercise. Heart rates are measured periodically and the cycle continues until all of the machines are utilized. A typical exercise session takes approximately 25 minutes to complete, but this time of exercise can be increased if desired.

The actual exercise intensity is determined by the participants themselves. Women that develop average exercise heart rates of from 110-120 per minute for the needed two hours per week will be developing a true CARDIO 120 program that can accomplish at least the first and possibly the good goal for cardiofitness.

A problem with the present Curves program and some other programs is the suggested maximum heart rate of 70% of so-called maximum for age. This limits both the effective cardio, health benefit and weight loss that can achieved by women over about age 60. This arbitrary percent of maximum heart rate is not valid for older persons. A heart rate of 110 to 120 beats per minute should be suitable for persons of all ages.

Many exercise experts feel that the Curves program is less intensive than they feel is needed. The resistance is fixed and is not raised stepwise, as in full resistance exercise. It also is true that if exercise heart rates are not increased adequately, the program will produce rather minimal benefits. But there seems to be a general agreement that this type of a program provides people a convenient and friendly way to initiate an exercise program.

Used as a CARDIO 120 program, the Curves protocol can provide the key aerobic exercise most needed for a healthy life. As women become more cardiofit, they can progress to more intensive resistance exercise programs if they wish. But the evidence we now have does not support a claim that higher levels of resistance training will contribute much more to long-range health.

The real key to health benefit from this type of a program is the actual exercise heart rates maintained. The Heart Method can compute from the Master Tables the likely cardio and health benefits from any intensity and time of exercise. Again, the Cardiofitness Point method can provide in a simple way the probable cardio benefits from this type of a program.

Music

As mentioned, exercise can be boring. The proper familiar music can help. Music is an inherent part of many exercise programs. Most younger people seem to use their iPod's when they exercise. Those older need to get some help from the younger in providing a way to enjoy music also. You can have music or the TV going as you exercise on a treadmill or exercise bicycle. Exercise programs on the TV usually play music. If you enjoy music of any kind, you should try to find a way to use it when you exercise

You Can Develop Your Own Exercise Program

Using a commercial gym or instructor-led program can be expensive. With an understanding of the Heart Theory of Exercise and Cardiofitness, you can design your own exercise program. For example, a mixture of fast walking and swimming such as I do could be useful. If you use a gym or buy exercise machines, you can set up your own combination of exercises. Although this book focuses on obtaining long-range health most efficiently, you may get most pleasure from a strong upper-body and want to concentrate exercise there. I then suggest that you try to accomplish this by developing a higher heart rate than usual during your exercise.

About Warm-up and Cool-down

The people that make exercise recommendations seem to assume that a person's time is of zero alternate value. We have present exercise recommendations for 3.5 and 7 hours per week of walking when no research available confirms that more than 2 hours per week can benefit health.

Nearly every exercise program recommends times for warm-up and cool-down. Some of this advice seems completely ridiculous. As example, an exercise program recommended by a supposedly prestigious university advises 5 minutes of brisk walking to be preceded by 5 minutes of slow walking and then followed by another 5 minutes of slow walking.

Can't we even walk briskly without preceding this by a full five minutes of slow walking? And then spending another five minutes cooling down? This might be useful for hospital patients that are just starting to walk again. But doing this does not seem even sensible for healthy adults. This could reduce the potential health benefits for the program of brisk walking by nearly three times.

Realistically our available time is not infinite. In the real world, 10 minutes of warm-up or cool-down time can be an alternate to 10 more minutes of good productive exercise. What value can we assign to warm-up and how does this compare with the health value of desirable exercise? How much warm-up do we really need to do?

It is claimed that warm-up heats up your muscles by increasing the movement of blood through your tissues; makes the muscles more supple; prepares your muscles for stretching; prepares your heart for exercise; helps prevent sport injuries; prepares you mentally; and prepares your nerves. It is also claimed that cool-down helps avoid fainting that results rarely from blood dropping to the legs after hard exercise; helps remove waste products from muscles and prepares your for the next exercise. I find nothing here about how warm-up reduced risk of major diseases or improved long range health. I found no research about risks of major disease encountered by those who did and who did not do warm-up from different types of exercise.

I spent many, mostly fruitless hours looking up and reading the research about warm-up. The research is unimpressive. An analysis of five studies concluded that "There is insufficient evidence to endorse or discontinue routine warm-up prior to physical activity to prevent injury among sports participants." Actually, three studies showed some small benefit, and two studies found no benefit. Some studies found some limited but unquantified benefit for warm-up; others found little or no benefit.[71]

But in no research study did I find any analysis of how much warm-up time is useful. Or a valuation of whether time spent in warm-up could be better spent in useful exercise. The research on warm-up was for athletes that did very vigorous exercise and that used quite long warm-up times. I have watched hundreds of people start to more moderate exercise. And only rarely did I see any of them doing much warm-up. I suspect that like so many dogmas about our health these warm-up times were derived long ago from speculation and then endorsed by endless repetition. There is a presumption that long warm-up times might make exercise safer and eliminate potential heart attacks. I find no research supporting this. If warm-up reduces potential useful cardiofitness development, it will most certainly increase and not reduce this risk.

It does seem sensible to start exercise carefully. As for example to swim the first few minutes of exercise at a lower level. Listen carefully for any signals your body gives that might involve a problem. But is it really productive to spend five or even ten full minutes doing this? The heart does its own warm-up. It takes about 3 minutes of exercise for it to reach a beating rate plateau at some exercise intensity. And it takes a full minute for it to reach half of this beating rate.

There have been instances where people fainted after very vigorous exercise probably because blood dropped down into lower blood vessels that were expanded due to very high-level exercise. exercise. It makes good sense to walk around for a while after strong exercise. But at this time I find no research that verifies when and how much time of this is really needed.

Keep in mind that most of the exercise for health suggested in this book and in CARDIO 120 is at the heart rates commonly obtained in very brisk to fast walking. If you do Managed Cardio at high heart rates, you should consider including some appropriate warm-up and cool-down procedure. It is sensible to start exercise slowly and work up to a desired intensity with reasonable care, and to walk around a bit after completing any vigorous exercise.

I make no recommendation about warm-up or cool-down except to cite what the research says. But more than sufficient research shows that up to two hours per week of useful cardio exercise has an important verified benefit in reducing risk of most important diseases.

Use the Life Ahead Computer Program

I have been developing the Life Ahead Program now for more than three decades. It now provides today's most comprehensive and sophisticated representation of how our lifestyle habits determine our risks of different major diseases, likely length of life, and the number of future days, both well and alive, we are likely to enjoy. The construct of the model and the health valuation of its included health factors are described and verified by nearly a hundred scientific papers provided on the www.lifeahead.net website

Appendix 6 tells how the program that is a free download from the internet values both cardiofitness and its health value. The program can compute how any amount of or change in various exercises will translate over time to cardiofitness in CFR, and how this in turn will translate into average Well-Days of life ahead. For example you can compute how any maintained change in pace and duration of walking, running, swimming, sports, etc. will change your likely Well-Days. Or how any combination of exercises such as swimming, aerobics, and weightlifting can contribute.

You can compute results for different exercise quickly from the demo program for a typical US population. But after entering you own risks and diet, you can develop a more accurate personal estimate how different exercises can provide benefits for you. The program also computes how nearly any change in diet or change in other major health risk factors will affect your risk of major diseases and change likely Well-Days ahead.

I hope that many of you that read this book will try out the Life Ahead Program. You can measure your cardiofitness from some different exercise machines and methods. And I will be pleased to hear about how the program worked for you and about any problems encountered. And I will welcome any suggestions for improvements.

CHAPTER 16

GETTING MOTIVATED TO EXERCISE CORRECTLY

Hundreds of health experts and doctors have been attending National Wellness Conference meetings at Stevens Point, Wisconsin for more that thirty years. They hear dozens of scholarly papers that focus on one key problem: How can we motivate people to care for their health? This is an enormously complex problem that has been and will continue to be a major problem of our society.

How I was Motivated

I was average-sedentary before participating in the company-sponsored exercise program. I thought I was in pretty good shape. The program taught me that I was not. There was no really good basis then for designing a personal exercise program. In trying to find out what I needed to do I found the research done even before 1980 to be overwhelmingly convincing about the importance of exercise. I learned then that I had a major need to exercise seriously and regularly.

I did do this exercise. But I was convinced of its importance only because I had done so much study of the actual research. I found no evidence that any others had studied this research in any depth. Most health researchers are focused on developing more and more new health studies for publication. Serious scientific analysis of what all research tells us on a subject can be very time-consuming and rarely is done.

The message about the benefits of exercise before about 1996 had remained controversial and confused. Despite 40 years of remarkably confirming research about exercise, some vocal researchers continued to demean its benefits until the Surgeon General Report of 1996 was published. After this, the opposition quieted and the health establishment finally moved consistently to advise people that "Exercise was good to do."

I've already mentioned my family history. Another motivation was what happened to some of my friends. During the single year I wrote my first book, four men of middle age that lived on two adjacent blocks dropped dead from heart attacks. A few years later we had dinner with another neighbor and his wife. The next morning his wife called in tears saying that her husband had died overnight. It was another heart attack.

If you do not now exercise, what can motivate you to exercise as described in this book? A poor health record in family history? Problems suffered by your friends? Does good exercise make you feel better and more alive? The pride of having a really fit body? The need to take off a lot of weight? Or are you just interested in doing everything possible to live a long and healthy life?

I Hope This Book Will Provide Motivation

This book was written to show the importance of proper exercise for health, and to help people get the best possible benefits from it. The book presents new findings that I hope will help motivate you to become and remain cardiofit.

1. The potential importance of cardiofitness to health. A very low cardiofitness can identify a higher risk of major disease and premature death than does any other major risk factor. It can identify risks of heart disease to 10 times, cancer to 4 times, and other important life-terminating diseases by 3 to 4 times. The magnitude of this risk seems to be near completely unknown to the public and to our health establishment. Cardiofitness is a physical condition of our heart and its associated cardiovascular system, the most important of all of our muscles.

2. Proper cardio exercise is the key – and the only key – that can reduce these large risks of poor cardiofitness. 85% of quantified risks of disease and health associated with exercise are due to and explained by cardiofitness. These facts endorse our cardio effective exercise as a most important thing most people can do today to live a life that is

184

both enjoyable and free of major disease. Diet can be similarly important, but most people today limit eating the important things that can make a diet very unhealthful. But most people today either do not exercise or do not exercise efficiently.

3. The new finding that a maximum cardio and health benefit from aerobic exercise is obtained from exercise of just two hours per week. Most past recommendations for exercise as for example of doing 30 minutes or an hour each day have been wrong. A vast amount of the time of our population is being wasted doing nearly useless amounts of exercise. This surprising two-hour limit throws a bomb at most previous ideas. It helps point us to the new Heart Theory of Exercise and Cardiofitness, which tells us what really happens. This knowledge can save us much wasted time.

4. A new approach developed for obtaining cardiofitness effectively and efficiently. Walking can produce useful cardiofitness but benefits depend sharply on pace. Walking at or below a usual pace can be ineffective. A new model shows for a first time how cardiofitness will develop from different maintained levels of cardio exercise heart rate and duration for men and women of all ages. Proper cardio-oriented exercise can develop benefits twice the potential from typical walking, and can reduce risk of heart disease by nearly four times.

A new Master Table method shows how exercise can be designed to produce a wide range of levels of cardiofitness from any kind or amount of cardio exercise. A new CARDIO 120 program shows how most people can obtain a first or good goal for cardiofitness and health from moderate levels of nearly any kind of exercise. The new concept of cardio feedback shows how a maintained CARDIO 120 might produce a very high level of cardiofitness from moderate exercise. A new Cardiofitness Point method shows those in exercise programs directly and simply how to exercise to desirable goals for cardiofitness and health.

5. The Cardiofitness Ratio, or CFR. This simple measure of our cardiofitness shows how our cardiofitness compares with others of our age. The CFR identifies the health value of our present exercise and related lifestyle. Most people, including many health professionals, have had little idea of the physical capability and fitness health risk of cardiovascular systems. We now can measure and monitor our actual level of cardiofitness in CFR from simple exercise tests.

6.   The importance of heart-rate-monitored exercise. Although strongly endorsed in the past, this major key to effective exercise and health management is being forgotten by most in today's health establishment The new technology shown in this book replaces those unfriendly and inaccurate 'percent of maximum heart rates' with simple direct heart rates we can easily measure.

Each increase of 10 beats per minutes in maintained exercise moves people toward a 50% higher level of cardiofitness. A carefully maintained moderate exercise heart rate not only can produce good levels of cardiofitness but can develop the cardio feedback that can develop very high levels of health protection. Without monitored heart rates, we may have no assurance that useful cardio benefit will be obtained from exercise. And without heart rate monitoring, the highly beneficial benefit of cardio feedback will not develop.

7.   The Heart Theory of exercise and cardiofitness. Cardiofitness identifies a physical condition of the heart and its cardiovascular system muscle that is improved by the same mechanism that improves muscle in resistance-type exercise. This gives you, as well as many experts, a better concept of how cardiofitness and its associated health benefits develop. It is not just the calories you burn or how long you walk that counts. It is how much the heart and its extensive cardiovascular system muscle is improved. An exercise that does not do this will not do much to improve our health.

The Heart Theory explains why that two-hour per week limit can occur for aerobic exercise. This newer understanding of how exercise produces its benefits can increase our confidence that doing the right exercise can produce real benefits to our cardiofitness and health. In the past the health benefits of exercise have been a near complete guess.

I also show how improving cardiofitness can improve the value of our exercise in reducing weight. I show that the fad of Step Counts can be a misdirection of the message needed to best help people. I suggest by example how the highest-intensity exercise done in just 2 hours each week can be far more important to the development of cardiofitness and health than are the remaining 112 hours of lower-intensity activity.

How Do US Adults Now Exercise?

An article about exercise in Time showed results of a poll that asked US people what exercise they now do every week. 69% claimed to walk regularly. Surveys by the NIH also confirm that 2/3rds of all people claim to walk for health. 35% say they use exercise machines, 30% say they ride a bike, 27% say they jog or run, and 22% say they do aerobic exercise. Many others claim other exercise such as hiking, golf, jog, and bowling. Only 21% admitted to not doing exercise.

I have considerable skepticism about these numbers. People inflate the frequency of doing things that are presumably good to do. Many respondents probably listed multiple entries because those citing jog or run also could cite aerobic exercise for the same exercise. The key question of how much of these exercises they actually do each week was not answered. But even if half of these numbers are valid, they show that many people probably now exercise regularly.

12% of the respondents cited their fitness (presumably cardiofitness) as excellent, and an incredible 69% listed themselves as "Fairly fit." Only 19% listed their fitness of "Not very fit or out of shape. This is fascinating because most people have had no useful way for identifying how fit they were. Realistically, about 50% probably were below average cardiofitness of 100 CFR.

Table 9-3 in Chapter 9 suggests that 20% of our population may be above the 120 CFR level of good cardiofitness, probably mostly from good aerobic exercise, and that another 16% are above the "Fair" level of 110 CFR. The remaining 64% have an important need to improve their cardiofitness.

Interestingly, more people claimed they were exercising for health than were exercising for weight. 83% of men and 86% of women cited "Improving health" as the key reason for exercising. 62% of men and 73% of women cited "Control of weight." 81% cited "Improving cardiovascular fitness." Thus most people have heard the message about exercise and cardiofitness. Yet few have had any very useful way for valuing what their cardiofitness means to health!

I found interesting the answers to "Do you enjoy your exercise." 72% said YES, only 21% said NO. These answers surprised me. But I was most pleased to see this, and I hope it is true.

Please review the Appendix items that follow. Some include guides and tables you should keep and use.

- *Appendix 1* provides four Master Tables. I hope you will copy these tables and keep them where they can be useful.

- *Appendix 2* describes in detail how to take the tests that measure your CFR.

- *Appendix 3* summarizes in more detail the surprising but extensive confirming research that shows that exercise of more than 2 hours a week provides healthy persons little if any further benefits to either cardiofitness or health.

- *Appendix 4* tells about maximum heart rates, and why these rates are useful only for identifying a highest desirable heart rate

- *Appendix 5* describes more formally the new Heart Theory of exercise and cardiofitness.

- *Appendix 6* tells how to use the Life Ahead #3 computer model to analyze your exercise and to estimate or measure your cardiofitness in CFR. The model will show how better cardiofitness from any kind and amount of exercise can reduce your risks of major disease and add more healthy days to your life.

- *Appendix 7* provides more of the remarkably convincing research that verifies the importance of cardiofitness.

APPENDIX 1

The Cardiofitness Master Tables

The Master Tables following show average improvements in cardiofitness expected for exercise of two hours per week, maintained at different exercise heart rates and heart rate elevations per week, for one year. Examples for using these tables were given in Chapters 4 and 5. Additional factors that modify the values from these tables for exercise of less than two hours a week and for months of exercise follow. More technical detail about the development of the Tables and the formulas involved is included following the Tables. The improvements in cardiofitness in CFR also will identify percentage improvements in a person's VO2 Max

CARDIO 120 Program and These Tables

A participant in this program needs only to maintain exercise heart rates in the range of 110 to 120 by any acceptable and useful exercise. The Master Tables confirm that this moderate exercise heart rate, when maintained for two hours each week, should produce useful improvements in cardiofitness for nearly everyone that is not now exercising regularly. Those with low resting heart rates of 80 or higher may have to use somewhat higher than listed exercise heart rates to obtain useful improvement in cardiofitness.

Table AP1-1

Table AP1-1 MASTER TABLES of CARDIOFITNESS Increase in the CFR from a starting level of 90 CFR for 2 hours/week exercise in one year								
Resting Heart Rate	50 or Less than 56		60 or 56 -65		70 or 66-75		80 or 76-80+	
Exercise Heart Rate Minutes 10 Seconds	Elevation in Heart Rate	Gain in CFR	Elevation in Heart Rate	Gain in CFR	Elevation in Heart Rate	Gain in CFR	Elevation in Heart Rate	Gain In CFR
70 12	20	4						
75 12	25	6						
80 20	30	8						
85 25	35	11						
90 15	40	13	30	7	20	2		
95 16	45	16	35	9	25	4		
100 17	50	19	40	11	30	6	20	2
105 18	55	22	45	13	35	8	25	4
110 18	60	25	50	15	40	9	30	5
115 19	65	29	55	18	45	11	35	7
120 20	70	32	60	21	50	13	40	8
125 21	75	36	65	24	55	16	45	10
130 22	80	40	70	27	60	18	50	12
135 23	85	44	75	30	65	21	55	14
140 23	91	48	80	33	70	23	60	16
145 24	95	53	85	37	75	26	65	18
150 25	100	57	90	40	80	29	70	20
155 26	105	62	95	44	85	31	75	23
160 27	110	66	100	48	90	34	80	25
165 28	115	71	105	51	95	38	85	28
170 29	120	76	110	55	100	41	90	30
175 30	125	82	115	59	105	44	95	33
180 30	130	87	120	64	110	48	100	36

The Master Tables can provide:

1. An estimate of an average improvement in cardiofitness from any amount or type of cardio exercise.

2. The design of a cardio exercise program to produce various target levels of cardiofitness improvement.

3. An estimate a person's genetic factor for cardiofitness.

Specific Instructions for doing these three steps follow: A low resting heart rate that identifies the zero point of exercise is needed for any of these estimates. Trainers that do not have this low resting rate can obtain an approximation by subtracting 5 beats per minute from a rate measured in an exercise facility.

1. How to Estimate an Average Cardiofitness Improvement in CFR from Regular Exercise:

    •   Get a measurement or best estimate of a usual exercise heart rate during exercise.

    •   Identify the column in the Master Tables that is nearest to the actual low resting heart rate.

    •   Read from the exercise heart rate in the left column over to the increase in CFR in the column for resting rate to identify a probable increase in CFR from this exercise. This provides an estimate for 2 hours per week of exercise for one year.

    •   If exercise is less than 2 hours per week, multiply the above value for CFR by the factor for time per week of exercise

    •   If exercise has been done for less than one year, multiply again by the factor for weeks of exercise.

    This will estimate the improvement in CFR that an average person would obtain from doing this level and amount of cardio exercise. This value for one year of exercise should be 10 CFR or more for a first goal, or 20 or more for the good goal of cardiofitness improvement. You now have a basis for estimating what changes would be needed to reach one or more of these goals. Improving cardiofitness will require a longer duration if duration is now less than 2 hours per week, or increase in exercise heart rate if duration is at the two hour per week limit. Some individuals may have genetic differences from average in the way their cardiofitness responds to exercise.

2. How to Design a Cardio Exercise Program to Reach a Goal for Cardiofitness:

    •   As in the first section above, identify the column nearest to the resting heart rate.

    •   Read down the column for increase in CFR to a desired value of increase in CFR.

    •   Suggest as a first goal an increase of 10 CFR, or a good goal increase of 20 CFR.

    •   Read over to exercise heart rate at a desired level. This identifies exercise heart rate to obtain a target CFR after a year of exercise of 2 hours per week.

- Check Appendix 4 to be sure heart rate estimated is below 90% of maximum heart rate. If not, a desired goal may not be achievable in one year. If heart rate is 120 beats per minute or lower, this step is not needed.

3. How to Estimate a Person's Genetic Susceptibility for Cardiofitness

- Estimate the individual's increase in cardiofitness from (1) above.

- If the individual is not physically active on the job or in general lifestyle, add the increase in cardiofitness from exercise to 90. This sum is an estimate of an average person's cardiofitness in CFR.

- Obtain a measurement of actual CFR as outlined in Appendix 2. Divide the estimated value by the actual CFR estimated and multiply by 100. This provides an estimate of cardiofitness genetic factor. If the value is less than 100, the person has a particular need to develop better cardiofitness from exercise than usual. This method may not be useful for persons that do substantial physical activity from work or lifestyle.

All values for exercise heart rates in these tables are averages of those of healthy individuals that have been medically approved for exercise and are doing exercise along accepted health guidelines. Actual values of improvement in CFR will vary somewhat for individuals that have different than usual response to exercise.

Heart rates in many exercise programs are taken for a time of only 10 seconds. Thus the corresponding 10-second values are noted in the tables. A 10-second rate of 20 indicates a minute rate of 120. This is a useful exercise heart rate for most healthy adults approved for exercise that usually is achievable after some modest level of cardiofitness is developed. If exercise is carried out at a measured exercise heart rate for periods up to several years, cardio feedback should improve cardiofitness to levels substantially higher than shown in these tables

The cardiofitness of levels of individuals can vary due to genetics. Individuals having a very low cardiofitness genetic factor, as for example values of 80 to 90, are advised that they have a serious risk factor associated with cardiofitness and have a particular need not only to develop a good cardio program but to pay particular attention to diet and all other health habits. But at this time the genetic factor method is developed from engineering analysis but has not been tested on an adequate number of people. I hope that researchers will test the method to verify that it usually will produce useful values.

If exercise duration is less than two hours per week, benefits are reduced as follows:

- 30 minutes: 29% of that at 2 hours 70 minutes: 66% of that at 2 hours

- 40 minutes: 33% of that at 2 hours 80 minutes: 76% of that at two hours

- 50 minutes: 48% of that at 2 hours 90 minutes: 86% of that at 2 hours

- 60 minutes: 57% of that at 2 hours 100 minutes: 92% of that at 2 hours

If exercise is done for periods of less than one year, multiply the table values to obtain a likely result for shorter times of exercise:

- 10 weeks: 0.4 times year value 30 weeks: 0.9 times year value

- 20 weeks: 0.75 times year value 40 weeks: 1.0 times year value

Heart stroke volumes used in developing the above tables are:

- 1.3 times at a 50 low resting heart rate

- 1.08 times at a 60 low resting heart rate

- 0.93 times at a 70 low resting heart rate

- 0 82 times at a 80 low resting heart rate

These values for stroke volumes are for information only. Do not use these factors in a computation.

The Master Tables And Their Development
(For Those Interested in Technical Details)

Exercise Energy from Exercise Heart Rates

The Master Tables provide what I believe is the first broadly useful and scientifically-based method for estimating how cardiofitness will develop from different levels of exercise heart rate maintained over time by men and women of all ages. More on the formulas and their statistical accuracy is included in the Life Ahead reference.[29] I have included here the actual formulas now used and a description of how this method was developed.

Cardiofitness develops from the higher flow rates of blood developed within the cardiovascular system that usually are generated from aerobic type exercise. These flow rates impart a stress in this system that is the counterpart of stress imparted to the arm muscles by weightlifting. A first question thus becomes, How does the energy that produces this stress develop from different blood flow rates in the cardiovascular system?

Chemical engineers know that the energy imparted to a flowing fluid usually moves up at the square, or 2nd power, of fluid flow rate at the general conditions present in the larger arteries of the cardiovascular system. This relationship is required to design the pump power needed to transfer different amounts of a fluid. The usual flow conditions in the pulsating cardiovascular system do not match those in the usual fixed conduits in engineering. But it still would be expected that energy imparted to the cardiovascular system by the flowing blood would develop at a power factor of the blood flow. This flow rate in turn is approximately proportional to exercise heart rate and heart rate elevation.

A study by Moon of the energy development from widely different exercise heart rates on a large population confirmed a sharply upward second power increase in energy as liters per minute of oxygen consumption with increase in heart rates above about 100 beats per minute.[36]

I tested the accuracy of different methods for measuring how cardiofitness from various measures of exercise intensity using the previously discussed database of 75 different results from 30 studies. These methods included percentages of maximum heart rate and a more involved method known as 'percentage of VO2 Max,' which is now used by most researchers. These other methods assume a direct proportional relationship between heart rates and energy that is not consistent with the expected power relationship. These researcher methods are useful for roughly identifying relative exercise intensity for a usual population of an average age. But they are not sufficiently accurate for inclusion in a broadly-based population model.

The simple heart rate elevation above resting heart rate at a given exercise duration proved to provide a better measure of cardiofitness development than did any of the above tested methods. A best relationship found between energy and cardiofitness was for the 1.6th power of heart rate elevation above low resting heart rate.

This confirms the likelihood from engineering and from the direct results of Moon that energy develops at a higher power of blood flow rate than unity. This explains in part why low-level increases in heart rate do not improve cardiofitness effectively.

Any inclusion of a maximum heart rate value in a formula for exercise intensity resulted in inaccurate valuations of cardiofitness development for people of different ages. This is because people of different ages develop cardiofitness similarly from a given elevation in heart rate. More on this in Appendix 4.

Development of the Master Tables

The Master Tables provide a mathematical model of the variables involved in producing blood flow rates, cardiovascular exercise, and improvements in cardiofitness. Eleven of these data sets that showed improvements in cardiofitness ranging from 20% to 47% were shown in Table 3-1. Results on both men and women were included about equally. Age levels ranging from 27 to 84 were represented, and results were included for from 10 to 52 weeks of exercise. It is of interest to explore the form of this mathematical model.

The actual formulas developed appear at the end of this Appendix. The predicted values represent improvements in cardiofitness expected for one year of exercise at the described conditions. These improvements were derived mostly from populations having an initial CFR level of about 90. But the values should be reasonable representative for adding to initial CFR values between 80 and 100.

The primary variable is the form dCFR = 0.0277 * (exercise heart rate − low resting heart rate) ^1.6 that identifies the effect of heart rate elevation above resting rate on the improvement in CFR as dCFR.

Factor 'a' adjusts for average hours per week of exercise if this is less than 2 hours. A maximum potential from exercise is taken as two hours per week.

Factor 'b' adjusts for no of weeks of exercise from start, with a maximum value as that at 50 weeks.

Factor 'c' adjusts for average heart stroke volume if resting heart rate is not 65. More on the significance of the formulas is included in the reference.[29]

The formula for the Heart Model of Cardiofitness follow as:

1. Increase in CFR from base = dCFR = (0.0277 * (hr - rhr) ^ 1.6) * a * b* c, where hr is exercise heart rate, and rhr is resting heart rate. This formula develops values for 50 continuous weeks of exercise, and assumes a 90 base level of CFR for a person that does little exercise. Those that do substantial physical activity, either in leisure or in occupation, can have higher base levels of CFR.

2. Adjustment of (1) for actual hours per week of exercise if less than 2. maximum Duration accepted is 2 hours. a is a value of 1.0 for two hours per week.

    a = 0.590 * hours/week - 0.0225 * hours/week ^ 3).

3. CFR loss for weeks of exercise less than 50 weeks.

    b is 1.0 at 50 or more weeks

    b = 0.00878 + 0.0437 * weeks - 0.00048*weeks^2.

    Maximum value is 50 weeks. Cardio feedback is not included.

    Minimum value for formula is 6 weeks.

4. Adjustment for stroke volume if low resting heart rate is not 65.

    c = 65 / low resting heart rate

    The highest values in the Master Tables can be extrapolations from this model that have not been directly confirmed by actual results.

APPENDIX 2

Measuring Your Cardiofitness

About These Tests

Three treadmill tests for cardiofitness Test A, Test B, and Test C are described here. A result from Test C is the basic test and is preferred. Test A and Test B use lesser intensities and provide only rough estimates of cardiofitness for those that are not reasonably cardiofit.

You should have a quality treadmill that can be set to various speeds in miles per hour and incline levels in percent. It should have a device for measuring heart rates. But you can develop the tests measuring your own heart rates if you wish. You should warm up for a few minutes at low intensity before starting any of the tests.

If you have been exercising regularly at measured exercise heart rates of 110 to 120 or higher, you should qualify to take Test C. You should not need to take the test sequence that follows and can skip to the entry following entitled "Test C is a Unique Test."

If you have not been exercising regularly, or are older or might be poorly fit, you should first take a sequence of these more moderate tests to identify which test is most suitable for you. An objective is to find which of three fitness tests will increase your heart rate into the 105 to 120 range.

Test A identifies a heart rate at a walking speed of 3.5 miles per hour and level incline that is designed to estimate the CFR of a man or woman of low cardiofitness doing a fairly brisk walk. First, at level incline set the speed to 2 or 2.5 miles per hour, and then warm up for a brief period. Move the speed up to 3.5 miles per hour either in one or two steps. If trouble is experienced walking at 3.5 miles per hour, you cannot take these tests. Your cardiofitness level is very low and you need to do more exercise for a few months before taking the tests.

The treadmill should then be set at the 3.5 miles per hour rate and level incline. If heart rates are not sufficiently elevated to near 120 beats per minute after three minutes of walking at this pace, the incline of the treadmill is raised to a 2% grade and heart rate measured for walking at the grade for Test B. If heart rates are not elevated close to 120 beats per minute after another two to three minutes of walking at Test B conditions, the pace and incline rates are reset to a 5% incline and 3.3 miles per hour for Test C. The heart rate after walking for 3 minutes in any test, but preferably that from test C, provides a basis for estimating cardiofitness in CFR.

If movement up to a higher load test produces a heart rate much above 120 beats per minute, the load should be moved back down and a result from the next lower level used henceforth or until cardiofitness becomes improved. Select the test for present and future use as the highest level test that produces heart rates close to but not much above 120 beats per minute.

The treadmill settings for the three treadmill tests are:

- Test A: Walk 3 minutes on treadmill set at 3.5 miles per hour and level grade (5.6 km/hr).

- Test B: Walk 3 minutes on treadmill set at 3.5 miles per hour and 2% grade (5.6 km/hr).

- Test C: Walk 3 minutes on treadmill set at 3.3 miles per hour and a 5% grade (5.2 km/hr).

Cardiofitness level in CFR can be estimated from a heart rate obtained in any of these tests using Table A2-1 for men or Table A2-2 for women. Be sure to use the Table values for the correct test method A, B, or C.

Test C is a unique test that, either as is or with some future improvements, should become part of a standardized method for cardiofitness testing. First, results from a similar test load are derived directly from the largest existing Cooper Institute database of 21,000 measurements of cardiofitness. Second, results from this test produce a direct estimate of the cardiofitness levels that produced results in this most respected research on the importance of cardiofitness to health and life.

I showed in Chapter 10 and in the scientific reference that the results at 5 minutes into the Cooper-Balke cardiofitness test were very highly correlated with results of the VO2 Max test, which is considered the best measure of cardiofitness. A person's heart rate after starting to exercise increases gradually to a plateau at any exercise load. Depending on the increase in heart rate obtained, this plateau is nearly always reached after three minutes of steady exercise at this load. This means that heart rates for 3 minutes into a simple treadmill fitness test should be similar to those at the 5 -minute time in the Balke test that used this same intensity of exercise.

Thus either the exact Cooper-Balke test done for only 5 minutes, or a simulation of this test via Test C proposed here, should provide a bridge between cardiofitness level and risk of major disease and death. No other known test for cardiofitness can provide this direct bridge between epidemiology research, cardiofitness level and health outlook.

About Taking the Cardiofitness Tests

It is best to take first fitness tests with the help of a fitness professional. And it always is desirable to take tests when others are with you. But you can take these tests by yourself. You always should take Test C if you qualify for this. But if you find from the above trial tests that Test A or Test B is best for you, take this test until your cardiofitness level improves. I will hope that those responsible in exercise facilities will be able to help people take these most useful tests. There are many other fitness tests, but none of these can usefully identify directly either the CFR or what their values mean for health. Some professional fitness tests also can be used to measure the CFR. More on this follows.

Developing a Value from Your Cardiofitness as CFR

Exercise for three minutes at the proper test speed and incline specified for your selected test. Read or take your exercise heart rate at this time. This is the only measurement you need to take from the test. Read a value for your cardiofitness in CFR from this heart rate as shown in Tables AP2-1 for men or AP2-2 for women following.

I suggest in Appendix 6 how to use the Life Ahead program, which can compute the results of these and other cardiofitness tests. This program can provide more information about how cardiofitness develops from various exercises and how your health benefits from better cardiofitness. (Download the program from www.lifeahead.net.)

Try taking your heart rate at one of the above treadmill test conditions on each of several days to see if you get the same result. An average of several test values may give the best result. You can do this as a part of your exercise program. But there are a number of things to keep in mind that can help you develop the most accurate results. Once you have some experience with the test, you can track over time how your cardiofitness changes with exercise .

Getting a Best Value for Your Cardiofitness

Your cardiofitness is measured from your exercise heart rate taken at some specified exercise load. A problem is that anything else you do that affects this heart rate also can affect the cardiofitness measurement. A resting heart rate usually is lowest during the morning before breakfast or any exercise. It tends to increase after each meal as the heart supplies energy for food digestion. It also can be elevated substantially due to exercise afterburn. This was shown in Figure 4-1 in Chapter 4.

Any factor that affects your resting heart rate also will similarly affect an exercise heart rate that is measured in a cardiofitness test. Thus it is best to take your exercise test at least 2-3 hours after food intake, before any exercise is done, and when you are not feeling poorly or are upset about something.

Your heart rate from an exercise test usually should be consistent within 1 to 2 beats per minute from tests taken on successive days. But if you are nervous or upset, this or many other things can affect your exercise heart rate. And keep in mind that exercise usually will improve the level of CFR by no more than 1 CFR each week. As before, you can obtain an average fitness test result.

About Accuracy

A change of just 1 in heart rate per minute will translate into a change in CFR of about 1.5 units. Thus a variation of plus or minus 2 in measured heart rate can mean a variation of plus or minus 3 units in cardiofitness.

You should be able to reproduce heart rates to within a usual 1-2 beats per minute. But this requires care in taking the test and in selecting the proper time of day to use it. Most people should try to obtain repeat measurements to refine the test reproducibility. It is best to take the test as part of an exercise program each week or month with recognition of the fact that actual levels of cardiofitness will change only slowly.

Values for Test A and B are estimated from exercise formulas and have not been directly verified.. But even if there is some bias in the CFR values computed from Tests A or B, the tests can be useful in approximating your cardiofitness, and should be able to track your progress. After your fitness improves, you may be able to take the more accurate Test C.

If you have exercise information measured as VO2 Max or wish to develop VO2 Max values from values of CFR, the formulas for doing this are shown following Table AP2-2. The reference values of VO2 Max for developing the CFR are provided in Table AP2-3. You also can estimate your CFR by dividing a VO2 Max value by the reference values given for age and gender in Table AP2-3.

It can be exciting to learn how your exercise heart rate goes down and your computed CFR improves as you continue your exercise. You learn that you can lift heavier weight and that your muscles are strengthened after doing resistance exercise. But there has been no available way for valuing the health benefit of aerobic type exercise except by taking an expensive and demanding VO2 Max test.

Getting a CFR from Other Fitness Tests

You can develop an estimate of your CFR from any fitness test that produces a value for VO2 Max. You can convert a usual VO2 Max value to a CFR using the equations following Table AP2-3. A caution is that the CFR does not vary for weight, and a VO2 Max value usually is adjusted for body weight. Thus this conversion will not be correct for individuals that differ much from average in body weight. You also can estimate a VO2 Max from a value of the CFR using the appropriate formula following Table AP2-2. The reference values for the CFR are shown in Table AP2-3.

If you have an actual result from a fitness test measured as VO2 Max, you can determine your CFR by dividing the VO2 Max value by a value from the following Table AP2-3 to obtain the CFR and then multiply this by 100. This table provides the reference or average population values used for the VO2 Max for those of different ages and gender. This conversion again is valid only for people of average or near average body weight. The CFR method and the Heart Theory of Exercise and Cardiofitness does not accept the theory that a change in body weight, as from diet, will have a true effect on the fitness of the cardiovascular system. Rather, cardiofitness is changed mostly by cardio-effective exercise.

Table AP2-1

Table AP2-1		For MEN			
Cardiofitness Ratio CFR for men from Cardiofitness Tests A, B, and C					
Test A 3.5 mph Level Incline		Test B 3.5 mph 2% Incline		Test C 3.3 mph 5% Incline	
Heart Rate	CFR	Heart Rate	CFR	Heart Rate	CFR
114	72	130	71	136	80
112	75	128	74	134	83
110	78	126	77	132	87
108	81	124	80	130	90
106	84	122	82	128	94
104	89	120	86	126	97
102	93	118	89	124	101
100	97	116	92	122	104
98	101	114	95	120	108
96	105	112	99	118	111
94	110	110	103	116	115
92	114	108	106	114	118
90	119	106	110	112	122
88	124	104	114	110	125
				108	129
				106	132
				104	136
				102	139
				100	143
				98	146
				96	150
				94	154
				92	157
				90	160

Table AP2-2

Table AP2-2		for **WOMEN**			
Cardiofitness Ratio CFR for Women from Cardiofitness Tests A, B, and C					
Test A 3.5 mph Level Incline		**Test B 3.5 mph 2% Incline**		**Test C 3.3 mph 5% Incline**	
Heart Rate	**CFR**	**Heart Rate**	**CFR**	**Heart Rate**	**CFR**
130	70	140	81	156	73
128	72	138	83	154	77
126	75	136	86	152	81
124	78	134	88	150	86
122	81	132	91	148	90
120	84	130	93	146	94
118	87	128	96	144	98
116	91	126	99	142	103
114	94	124	102	140	107
112	98	120	105	138	111
110	101	118	109	136	116
108	105	116	112	134	120
106	109	114	116	132	124
104	113	112	120	130	129
102	117	100	123	128	133
100	122	98	127	126	137
98	126	96	132	124	141
				122	146
				120	150
				118	154
				116	158
				114	163

The formulas used for deriving the CFR from values of VO2 Max are:

- For Men: CFR = VO2 Max * 100 / (33.0 + (50 - age)*0.24

- For Women: CFR = VO2 Max * 100 / (25.3 + 50 − age) * 0.18)

- From CFR to VO2 Max

- For Men: VO2 Max = CFR * 0.01 * (33.0 + (50 - age)*0.24)

- For Women: VO2 Max = CFR * 0.01 * (25.3 + (50 − age)*0.18)

Table AP2-3

CFR Reference Values of VO2 Max		
Age	Men	Women
20	40.2	30.7
30	37.8	28.9
40	35.4	27.1
50	33.0	25.3
60	30.6	23.5
70	28.2	21.7
80	25.8	19.9
90	23.4	18.1

APPENDIX 3

Two Hours a Week of Aerobic Exercise is Enough

This conclusion is near certain to invite controversy. Obviously, we need abundant evidence to accept that there is little or no additional cardio or health benefit from aerobic exercise of more than two hours each week. I initially was highly skeptical about this finding. As more and more confirming evidence became available, I studied the available data exhaustively looking for flaws.

There now is abundant and overwhelming evidence that shows that more than about two hours per week of aerobic exercise produces only minimal additional benefits to health. I find no useful evidence supporting the reverse hypothesis that aerobic exercise at a given intensity done for more than two hours per week can be of useful value to cardiofitness or health for non-diabetic persons of healthy weight.

This section reviews the research in more detail than was done in Chapters 2 and 3. The actual research data and further analysis of walking is provided in the internet reference.[20] The research data and the analysis of cardiofitness development from differing durations of exercise also is provided.[29]

The finding of this two-hour limit for benefits from aerobic exercise evolves from Global Scientific Analysis. It was only when results of all studies were analyzed together to identify the causal effects of walking pace and duration that the conclusion emerges both sharply and with high significance. This result would not have been evident from any single study, and would not have been found by a conventional statistical meta-analysis.

I suggest in Appendix 5 that an upper limit for effective exercise also applies to usual resistance exercise. The gain in strength for three such exercise sessions per week may be only marginal vs. that from just two sessions per week. Further, there seems to be no gains in muscle from doing more than three resistance exercise sessions per week.

The limiting time of stress for effectiveness of resistance exercise may be much less than the two hours per week limit for aerobic exercise. The Heart Theory holds that both aerobic and resistance exercise derive their benefits from what is essentially resistance exercise. Both exercises develop muscle. Thus there appear to be clear limits to the duration of exercise that can be effective in improving muscle.

Risks of Heart Disease from Walking

Table AP3-1 shows results from all of the useful studies I could find relating risks of heart disease to various durations of walking at consistent intensity.

I first ran conventional meta-analyses of the separate effects of walking duration and walking intensity on risk of disease. The effect of walking intensity was highly significant and consistent and showed a strong relation between walking pace and risk of disease. But the effect of walking duration on risk of disease was small and only barely significant. There did appear to be benefits for shorter duration exercise, but the longer exercise showed no further benefit.

It was obvious that the meta-analysis for exercise duration was meaningless. There was an effect of exercise for short periods, but none for successively longer periods. This was troubling because all recommendations about exercise stressed substantial durations. There was a need to examine the research in more detail.

Note that some of the research in Table AP3-1 are not ordinary studies. Four are today's largest available and now classic studies of populations of 39,000 to 72,500 men and women. *Study #1* showed a 35% reduction in risk for nearly 6 hours of exercise. This is not significantly higher than the 30% reduction developed from two hours of exercise. *Study #2* show the same reduction in risk for durations of more than 2 hours than for much shorter durations. *Study #3* showed little effect of duration on benefits. *Study #4* showed essentially the same benefits for 4 hours as for 2 . Both men and women in *study #6* showed no advantage for a twice higher 5 hours than that for just 2 hours.

Study #5 identified results per day rather than per week, and included no value for the important two hour per week time. It showed a confusing benefit for the small difference between 3.5 hours a week and 5.3 hours, but no added value for 10 hours vs. 5.3 hours. These confusing results do not contribute a useful addition to this analysis.

The results of *study #7* of the mail carriers found nearly the same benefits as those obtained in other studies for walking just 2 hours per week. Mail carriers typically walk 10 miles per day or more, or 30 hours per week. They also carry a heavy bag. Their estimated 4,000-5000 calories of physical activity per week produced similar benefit

Table AP3-1

Table AP3-1 Effect of Walking Duration on Risk of Heart Disease			
Study	Walking Duration Hours/Week	% Reduction in Risk of Heart Disease	Results
1. Manson, 72,500 Women Nurses	2.2	30	No
	5.9	35	Significant Difference
2. Lee, 39,000 Women's Health Professionals	1-1.5	51	No
	over 2	52	Significant Difference
3. Tanasescu 44,500 Men Health Professionals	avg 0.9-1.8	-3	No
	7.2 hours	10	Significant Difference
4. Manson, 73,000 women's WHI	2.1	46	No
	4.0	39	Significant Difference
5. Noda, 42,000 men in Japan	3.5	24	No values
	5.3	46	at 2 hrs/wk,
	10	42	No
Noda, 31,000 women in Japan	3.5	50	benefits for
	5.3	72	10 vs 5.3
	10	76	hrs/wk
6. LaCroix, 1650 men in Canada	2.5	22	No
	5	11	Significant Difference
Same for Women	2.5	50	No
	5	55	Significant Difference
7. Morris and Kahn, Mail Carriers vs usual Results for Walking	2	56	No
	30	50	Significant Difference

to those developed by other groups that walked only a few hundred calories per week. This is one of the many research results that show that calories of exercise can contribute little to either risk of disease or cardiofitness. The study US of mail carriers by Kahn showed that only the carriers that walked and delivered mail obtained benefits. Benefits were lost by the carriers that transferred to office jobs.

Most of the individual researchers did point out that pace was more important than duration. But what now appears evident from the review of all studies was not sufficiently evident in the individual studies to arouse the attention of researchers.

As a further test I combined the results of all of the available comparisons of walking risk and walking duration from the available useful studies in order of hours walked per week.[20] Some of these results were mentioned in Chapter 5. The more complete results:

For walking of about one hour per week, average risk of heart disease was reduced by 23%. For walking to 2 hours per week, average risk of heart disease was reduced by 38%. This means that the 2nd hour per week of walking produced 15% added benefit vs. the 23% of the first hour.

But for walking to 3 hours per week, average reduction in risk was a lower 34%, or no more than the 38% for two hours of walking.

For walking 5 hours per week: No further benefit for walking more than 2 hours per week.

For walking ten hours per week, same conclusion.

For the mail carriers, there was little further benefit from perhaps 30 hours per week of walking.

Formulas and some significance values are in the referenced paper.[20]

An important qualification of this two hour per week limit for benefit is that this refers to durations of walking at the same pace and same exercise intensity. Some studies showed larger benefits for longer periods of exercise, but this also involved higher exercise intensity for those that exercised longer times. Some studies related statistical associations of risk to estimates of calories, METs (metabolic equivalent tasks) or and MET-hours and did not report actual durations of exercise. These associations are not usefully casual or valid. I had to estimate the probable amounts of exercise duration from these studies.

The only useful result that did not confirm the two hour limit was that for a subset of women that had diabetes in the above Nurses' Health Study.[73] Diabetics have an extremely high risk associated with weight, BMI, and blood sugar. It is not surprising that more walking hours than usual could improve their risk. But the much larger total groups of healthy women in the same study did not benefit either in risk of heart disease or in all-cause mortality from walking more than two hours per week.

Risks of Death from All Causes is Reduced by Only Two Hours Per Week of Walking

There is further evidence from the large Nurses Study that this same two hour per week limit applies to risks of death from all causes. A study of Rockhill shows that no further reduction in risk of death from cancer or from all causes occurs for groups walking more than 3 hours per week (probable average 4-5 hrs/week) than those walking an average of 2 hours per week.[74] Keep in mind that this is a very large study, and that 4-5 hours is more than twice 2 hours.

With such a large difference as a doubling in exercise duration we would expect a large difference in benefit. We see none. The risk of death from all causes involves a risk of that is a much more important than is the risk heart disease developed by most other studies.

The Limit of Two Hours per Week also Applies to the Development of Cardiofitness

This finding provides the key to why the risk of disease did not decline for higher durations of exercise. Benefits for risk of heart disease from exercise derive mostly from improvements in cardiofitness. It appears that the failure of more than two hours per week of exercise to improve health benefits is due to the fact that more than that does not improve cardiofitness further.

A study by Ready[34] tested similar groups of women that walked the same hour program 3 and 5 days per week. The 3-day group gained 12 in CFR; the 5-day group gained 13 CFR – an insignificantly different benefit from an initially somewhat less fit group. If fitness progressed as normally would be expected, the CFR of the 5-day group should have advanced to a 20 or higher CFR.

A large of study of 350 persons by Hellerstein[75] found that those who trained between 2.2 and 3.0 30-minutes sessions per week did better than those training 1-2 sessions per week. But those training 3.5-5.0 sessions per week obtained no further benefit over those training 2-3 per week.

A study in Japan of Step Counts described in Chapter 14 found that groups of both men and women of different ages all obtained an improvement in cardiofitness of about 9% from an added estimated 6 hours of probable walking each week. This is the same improvement in cardiofitness that would be obtained for 2 hours per week of typical brisk walking.

The 75 results of cardiofitness improvement from exercise also were organized in order of their duration in hours per week.[29] The increase in CFR was then forecast for one year of exercise from all factors except duration. This method produced an estimate of the effect of duration from each comparison. The accuracy of this estimate was improved by taking an average from multiple values in different ranges of exercise duration in hours per week.

The value for durations of 0 to 0.99 hours per week – at an average duration of 0.65 hours – showed a benefit value of only 0.36. At 1.5 hours per week the effect of duration had advanced to 1.07, and at an average of 2 hours the value of duration reached 1.29. The values for duration of exercise from 2 to 2.9, 3 to 3.9 and 4+ hours per week showed no significant further benefit beyond the value for 1.5 to 2.5 hours of exercise of 1.29 per week A value of 1.00 in this analysis represents a value of exercise done for 24 weeks.

The above results are for averages of up to 26 individual research comparisons in each time period. If the benefit for exercise duration in hours per week had progressed in a more normal and expected way, the duration value for 3-3.9 hours per week should have been 2.25, and the value of 4+ hours per week would have been at least a value of 3.00 Actual values were only 1.39 and 1.07, respectively.

This analysis shows that cardiofitness did improve for exercise of up to about 2 hours per week. But it did not improve further after this time of exercise was exceeded. Differences in cardiofitness are the primary factor that produces differences in risk of heart disease. The reason for the failure of more exercise than this to provide benefits to heart disease is that cardiofitness does not improve for exercise of more than this 2 hours per week. This behavior produces further confirmation of the important link between cardiofitness level and risk of heart disease.

This Finding of a limiting benefit for Exercise Is of Importance Is Very Significant

A usual reaction of some health researchers is to quickly dismiss surprising findings like this, saying "This is controversial. We need more research to confirm this." The finding here is that more than two hours per week of aerobic exercise at a given exercise intensity does not usefully improve either cardiofitness or heart health. This is for those that are healthy and not overweight or obese. My answer here is that we do not need any more research to confirm this finding.

The research data we now have for walking and risk of heart disease include results from a combined population of more than 450,000 persons. Four of the nine useful studies were done on from 29,000 to more than 72,000 men and women. Available research includes durations of exercise ranging up to 30 hours per week. The confirming research includes our largest and most respected health studies. The results from this research on walking are confirmed by results from 75 data sets on cardiofitness development from different kinds and durations of exercise. Cardiofitness similarly is not improved by more than 2 hours per week of aerobic exercise of a given intensity.

The same finding emerges from multiple results on exercise duration and heart disease and exercise duration and cardiofitness. The fact that the same duration for effective exercise was found in two entirely separate families of evidence greatly increases the casual likelihood of its validity. This confirmation further supports the importance of cardiofitness as a key risk of heart disease.

The chance that much more research of this magnitude and scope will become available in the foreseeable future is remote. The chance that a multiplicity of research will become available that could challenge or change the overall result from this large database in the foreseeable future is close to nil.

The actual results of this research are organized and provided in the referenced study. Anyone is free to analyze the data in this table or refine it or add data to it. Science requires an explanation that fits all of the available research. This is what has been done here. And I find no useful or significant research now published that provides an opposing conclusion.

Turning the Hypothesis Around

A logical requirement in view of this finding would be to test the hypothesis that there is a useful benefit to health and cardiofitness for exercise of more than two hours per week. Asking an entire population to spend billions of hours doing exercise from evidence that cannot pass this test does not seem appropriate.

I could not find any evidence on healthy people that would pass this test. I would think that any responsible group that advises the public about their exercise should be able provide a published basis that both recognizes the research cited herein and confirms at high statistically accuracy this alternate hypothesis.

How Accurate Is This Two Hour Limit?

A limit of exercise duration for cardiofitness development is consistent with and forecast by the Heart Theory of Exercise and Cardiofitness. Within the accuracy of the information now available, the limit could be as low as 1.75 hours – or a bit more than two hours. There might still be rather small additional benefit for longer exercise than this two hours per week. It is possible that there could be a limit to how much cardiofitness and muscle could be improved in a single exercise session, or in one day. The effect of exercise on serum cholesterol probably will continue to reduce risk after the 2-hour limit. But the magnitude of this benefit as shown in Table 8-1 is small.

The first hour of walking may produce at least 60% of the benefit of two hours. The limit could be different for exercise at much higher exercise intensities. Competitive runners train at many hours per week to obtain maximum fitness. They may be spending much of this time gaining only a very small improvement in cardiofitness, but this small amount could be the key to winning. This finding raises questions about training for competition. How much do extra hours beyond two per week in training at a controlled exercise intensity really help in improving cardiofitness and race times? Research to test this at athletic levels of intensity would be of considerable interest.

I estimate that 1.5 hours per week of exercise produces 86% of the benefit of two hours per week. As I have discussed elsewhere, it seems reasonable to suggest a program of 1.5 hours per week of direct aerobic exercise if a person also does some resistance exercise that usefully increases exercise heart rate. And to the extent resistance exercise can be developed to produce more aerobic exercise, this time for associated direct aerobic exercise can be reduced further. The aerobic exercise contribution of resistance exercise to cardiofitness now can be estimated by measuring average heart rate elevations developed during this exercise together with the Master Tables and method described in Appendix 1.

APPENDIX 4

About the Maximum Heart Rate

Nearly every recommendation about exercise and heart rates has been to exercise at some percentage of maximum heart rate. A high percentage value as 85% to 90% of maximum heart rate can be a useful guide for the maximum heart rate that should be used in exercise by those accustomed to vigorous exercise. But modern research shows that exercise at similar actual exercise heart rates produces similar improvements in cardiofitness for men and women of all ages. Estimates of desirable exercise heart rates based on percentages of maximum heart rate can be seriously incorrect.

The Maximum Heart Rate

Most physical functions of the human body tend to decline with age after our 20's or 30's. One of these functions is the maximum rate at which a heart will beat. This maximum beating rate usually starts at a bit above 200 in youth and declines about seven to ten beats per minute each succeeding 10 years. This appears to be a physiological control or pacemaker in the body that avoids over-exercising the heart.

Maximum Heart Rate as a Useful Guide

It was learned more than a half-century ago that the maximum heart rate usually declines with age and follows roughly a simple formula of 220 minus age. It also was well known that exercise at high heart rates was much more effective for producing cardiofitness than was exercise at low heart rates. The maximum heart rate was a ceiling heart rate, and it seemed logical that exercise somewhat below this highest rate, at say 85% to 90% of maximum, was a desirable and highest prudent level for exercise.

There was no useful research then relating cardiofitness to risks of disease, but it seemed likely that exercising at these high heart rates would be most beneficial. The public owes a debt to the remarkable forecasts of Dr. Samuel Fox, Kenneth Cooper and other early exercise experts about how exercise produces its benefits. Their forecasts were made three decades before direct research verifying the value of cardiofitness was actually published. Millions of middle-age and younger people that did productive heart-rate-monitored exercise probably improved cardiofitness substantially, extended their lives and contributed to the enjoyment of better health.

Percentages of Maximum Heart Rate
Do Not Produce Useful Values for Exercise Intensity

A high percentage, as for example 85% or 90%, of maximum heart rate can produce a useful basis for a highest exercise heart rate to use. But a serious problem of bad mathematics occurred when people started using lower percentage values of this maximum heart rate as measures of exercise intensity and for recommending heart rates for exercise.

Heart rate does not go to zero with zero exercise. It moves down only to resting heart rate. At age 80 for example, a usual resting heart rate for zero exercise becomes 54% of a calculated maximum heart rate. People were using a system that implied that a 54% of maximum heart rate meant 54% of maximum exercise. More accurately, a 54% of maximum heart rate could mean exercise at resting heart rate, *or zero exercise*. In fact, percents of maximum heart rate such as 50%, 60% and even 70% can have virtually no useful meaning for exercise intensity for those of different ages, and were most seriously in error for older people.

Yet despite these flagrant mathematical errors, percents of maximum heart rate still continue to be implied as something 'scientific.' We see these numbers of "percentage of maximum heart rate" still posted in exercise facilities as maximum desirable heart rates for men and women of different ages. Such numbers can be misleading mathematical garbage.

These errors were recognized and corrected long ago by researchers by use of a method called 'heart rate reserve' and other methods. These methods recognized that zero exercise was at resting heart rate. But the misleading numbers of percentage of maximum heart rate for exercise intensity and for prudent heart rates continue to be presented to the public to this day. Heart rates commonly proposed of say 50% to 60% of maximum really identify near zero exercise for older people.

There is another problem with use of the maximum heart rate. A common practice in recommending exercise heart rates has been to specify a range of say 50-85% of maximum heart rate. The theory here was that this identified exercise heart rates that were useful for conditioning the body. This was not true.

As example, for the estimated 170 maximum heart rate at age 50, this suggests a rate of from 85 to 145 beats per minute. The Master Table 5-2 shows that each 10 beat difference in exercise heart rate maintained over time is quite important to cardiofitness. An exercise heart rate of 85 is much too low to produce cardio benefit. This recommendation thus has little real usefulness. A level of at least 75% of maximum heart rate is needed at age 80 to effectively develop even minimal cardiofitness.

These recommendations about how to exercise at different percents of maximum heart rate suggested exercise at 3 to 5 times per week of 15 to 60 minute durations. This endorses from 45 minutes to 300 minutes per week as presumably recommended times for exercise. This overly wide range of heart rates and durations again produces little guidance to someone that wishes to know how to exercise. Research now shows that more than 120 minutes of exercise per week will be of little value to health.

Maximum Heart Rate Values Are Not Accurate

Another problem is that the usual formula of maximum heart rate equals 220 minus age is not accurate. A more accurate formula called the Miller formula is: Maximum heart rate = 217 minus 0.85 times age. A study of 43 different published formulas for predicting maximum heart rate concluded the best one was 205.8 minus 0.685 times age. The penalty for age used in the usual formula appears to be much too high, and produces much lower than probable safe and needed exercise heart rates for older people.

Recommendations of the ACSM and AHA suggested the use of exercise heart rates up to 90% of maximum rate. Heart rates at maximum and at 90% of maximum for the most accurate formula are shown in Table AP4-1. These rates are useful only for healthy people that are accustomed to vigorous exercise.

Table AP4-1

Heart Rates for Most Accurate Formula: Maximum HR= 205.8 – 0.685 Times Age						
Age	30	40	50	60	70	80
Maximum Heart Rate	185	178	172	168	158	151
90% of Maximum	167	160	155	149	142	136

This best formula still had a standard error value of +/- 6.4 beats per minute. This means that for a 180 maximum heart rate the 5% to 95% range of individual rates would be from 159 to 203 beats per minute. The maximum heart rate thus is a very inaccurate number. Even using the 'best' formula, an actual maximum heart rate can vary 44 beats per minute for different persons of the same age. Further, a maximum heart rate can vary 3-5 beats per minute depending on measurement by treadmill or bicycle, or by treadmill walking or running. So any formula value for a maximum heart rate provides only a very rough estimate of a true value.

The CARDIO 120 method and most advice in this book call for moderate exercise that will be well below maximum heart rates computed from any of these formulas. Only those that exercise at rather high heart rates and who are athletic, or those older and quite fit probably will need to be concerned about their maximum heart rates. The Heart Method of Exercise and Cardiofitness does not use this very inaccurate maximum heart rate method in assessing intensity of exercise.

Maximum Heart Rate Should Not Be Included in a Recommendation for Exercise Intensity

As before, research now suggests that a given heart rate elevation during exercise will produce the same or at least similar improvement in cardiofitness for those of differing ages. Thus recommendations about heart rates needed for useful gains in cardiofitness should not include any modifier for age. Any use of a maximum heart rate in advice on how to exercise inserts a large modifier for age that has no valid basis.

Resting Heart Rates Also Are Important

Another problem with the conventional use of maximum heart rates is that no consideration is given to the important factor of resting heart rates The resting heart rate of individuals can vary from below 50 to above 90 beats per minute. Thus resting rate can have a major effect on true exercise of the heart and development of cardiofitness at a given exercise heart rate.

This is illustrated by the Master Tables of exercise intensity described in Appendix 1. For example, a heart rate of 120 for a person having a resting rate of 50 will produce a very large gain of 32 CFR. This same heart rate for a person with an 80 resting heart rate will produce a 4 times lower gain of only 8 CFR.

It is heart rate elevation and not just heart rate per se that produces the flow of blood that exercises the heart and its cardiovascular system cardiofitness. An athlete with a low resting heart rate of 40 will gain more true exercise of the cardio system at an exercise rate of 80 beats per minute than will a person have an 80 resting rate will achieve at an exercise rate of 160 beats per minute.

When I was measured at a CFR of 150, my low resting heart rate was 49. Walking nearly 5 miles per hour and moving into jogging failed to increase my heart rate above 85 beats per minute. An average person would obtain exercise heart rate of 120 to 130 with this exercise. Good athletes can have resting heart rates in the low 40's. They can develop substantial cardio blood flow at a heart rate of only 70 beats per minute.

Most physiologists have abandoned the percentage of maximum heart rate method for estimating exercise intensity and use a better method called percent of VO2 Max. This method gives a rough measure of exercise intensity for individuals of one specific average age that is useful for a specific research study.

But this percentage of VO2 Max method is too involved for individuals to use. The method also undervalues high heart rate exercise because the analysis from 75 study comparisons shows that effective exercise increases as the 1.6 power of heart rate elevation. And the percentage of VO2 Max method also involves the inaccurate maximum heart rate that identifies a relative exercise intensity for age, and not the actual levels of intensity that are needed for assessing health benefits for those of different ages.

The Heart Theory Method Produces Simple and More Accurate Valuations

The Heart Theory of Exercise and Cardiofitness uses the simple heart rate elevation selected as in Master Table 5-2 and Appendix 1 that applies usefully to people of all ages and gender. This forecasts directly how much cardiofitness will develop from a specific heart rate elevation maintained for identified periods of time.

The key that produces cardiofitness is exercise of the heart and its cardiovascular system. This exercise is produced by the amount of pulsing blood flow that is pushed through the cardiovascular system. The amount of this blood is quantified in part by the elevation in heart rate above the rate it beats at rest. If exercise heart rate is 110, and resting rate is 70, our elevation is 40. This simple number provides most of what we need to know to understand how cardiofitness develops. This model develops directly from engineering fundamentals and physical science.

At a value of zero elevation in heart rate the low resting heart rate supports only our basal metabolism. Our physical exercise raises the heart rate above this metabolic, or minimum, rate. Useful cardiofitness development for an average person starts at an elevation in exercise heart rate of about 30-35 beats per minute above metabolic rate. Elevations of 40, 50, and 60 are the values most people will need to use to improve cardiofitness effectively. Each increase in maintained exercise heart rate provides a higher potential level of cardiofitness.

A measure commonly used in physiology is METs. One MET identifies the energy required to support our basal metabolism. Thus our low resting heart rate identifies one MET of energy at zero exercise. As our heart rate increases above its low resting rate, the number of METs of energy will increase. A value of 7 METs is often used to describe a useful level of cardio energy. Values of 9 to 10 METs represent a high level of cardio exercise. Just two METs will not produce useful cardiofitness.

The present Heart Method estimates a person's VO2 Max from exercise heart rates and time of exercise. The CFR is the ratio of this estimated Value of VO2 Max to average for age and gender. A common relationship is that VO2 Max equals 3.5 times mets in ml/kg/min. Thus the CFR could alternately be taken as a ratio of an actual value of METs to usual METs for age and gender because the Heart Method effectively also measures a value of METs. But using METs per se as a measure encounters the same problems that make the VO2 Max method useless to people as a measure of cardiofitness. The value changes significance substantially with people's age and gender.

In Conclusion

High percentages as 85% to 90% of maximum heart rate are useful for identifying a likely maximum heart rate for prudent exercise of individuals that are accustomed to doing vigorous exercise. Lower percentages of maximum heart rate than this do not provide useful values for either exercise intensity or prudent heart rates for people of different ages. The maximum heart rate also is an inaccurate number that should not be used in a recommended measure of exercise intensity The use of actual exercise heart rate and resting heart rate will produce results that are both much more accurate and much easier to use.

APPENDIX 5

The Heart Theory of Exercise and Cardiofitness

A Serious Question is, How Does Physical Activity Protect Our Health?

We now have thousands of studies about physical activity. Physical activity can benefit health in many different ways. There has been endless speculation about possible contributing factors. Yet to my knowledge we have no quantified scientifically-based explanation of how physical activity produces health benefits as was done in Chapter 8..

Researchers have been studying exercise and cholesterol for many years. Yet this and other related factors, when quantified, turn out to be close to trivial when compared with the far larger effect on health that is related to cardiofitness. I have seen no clear quantitative verified identification of what 'physical activity' accomplishes in the body beyond that which more accurately relates of cardiofitness.

The words 'physical activity' identify all kinds of physical activity. They include physical activity in the household, office, on that job and that from activities we call exercise. The major focus of much of our research establishment had been on physical activity. The title of the Surgeon General's report was "Physical Activity and Health." Textbooks about exercise use this title, and most books on exercise have not usefully identified the role and importance of cardiofitness.

Cardiofitness is quite different from ordinary physical activity or exercise. Cardiofitness is a measurable physical condition of the heart and its cardiovascular system that is produced only by certain kinds and amounts of exercise. The exercise that produces cardiofitness best is aerobic, or cardio exercise. This does not have to be extremely high-intensity exercise. But intensive exercise produces the highest levels of cardiofitness.

Physical activity is usually measured as energy calories. We have more than enough evidence that shows that calories of energy are not primary in producing cardiofitness. . Postal carriers get little more from large amounts of walking than do others that walk two hours per week. Those in heavy physical occupations that exert thousands of calories per day obtain no more benefit than do those that just walk a reasonable amount.

Why is this true? I noted in Chapter 1 that Blair obtained at least five times the health benefit from fewer calories of cardio exercise than did Paffenbarger from ordinary calories of physical activity.

Research on cardiofitness does explain this part of the problem. Only physical activity of certain durations and sufficient intensities will usefully improve the fitness of the cardio system. Most physical activity is not of sufficient intensity or duration to do this and thus does not produce effective cardiofitness improvement.

The key importance of cardiofitness is that it explains how exercise reduces the risk of diseases far more accurately than does any other measure of physical activity. Improved cardiofitness reduces or probably reduces risk of cardiovascular disease, most or all types of cancer, diabetes, dementia, macular degeneration, COPD, arthritis, nephritis and osteoporosis. Cardiofitness can identify differences in risk of major disease up to several times more effectively than does any general measure of physical activity.

The puzzling questions then become, How can cardiofitness that is a direct measure of muscle capability in the cardiovascular system reduce the multiplicity of above disease risks? How does this measurement of muscle improvement selectively protect against diseases that involve widely different and complex biochemical processes throughout the body? These factors of cardiovascular muscle capability and multiple biochemical processes throughout the body appear disparate.

We also have another puzzling finding to explain. Why does exercise of more than about two hours each week produce little or no further benefit to cardiofitness and risk of major disease? The evidence about this is extensive.

The Heart Theory of Exercise and Cardiofitness

The Heart Theory that follows appears to explain most of these puzzling findings. It offers a tenable theory of why cardiofitness can be more concisely related to risk of disease than is any other factor. It explains why given calories of exercise may produce good or very little health benefit. It explains why exercise intensity and not energy calories is the key to cardio and health benefit. It explains quantitatively how health benefits can derive from different amounts and intensities of exercise. And it explains why there can be a two hour per week limit to the amount of exercise that protects health.

The heart uniquely exercises itself 24 hours each day at about 70 times each minute and a hundred thousand times every day. Each beat of the heart pushes blood into the aorta and into some thousands of miles of arteries, capillaries and other vessels throughout the entire body. When at rest, the heart may beat at a somewhat relaxed rate. But once it reaches about 25-30 beats per minute above its resting rate, it usually operates like most other pumps that move an equal amount of fluid with each stroke.

As heart rate increases, the increased flow of blood places more and more stress on all vessels throughout the cardiovascular system. This includes pushing open those crucially important coronary arteries that usually are involved in heart disease, as was impressively demonstrated by Figure 7-3. This higher flow of blood through thousands of miles of blood vessels nourishes all contacted blood vessels better with its dozens of included nutrients. The increased energy and pressure from increased blood flow exercises the pulsating heart and other vessels in the cardiovascular system.

A tenet of the Heart Theory is:

The flow rate of blood in the cardiovascular system developed by exercise provides a level of exercise stress. A duration as two hours per week of a highest usual level of this stress develops cardiofitness.

Cardiofitness Develops from Resistance Exercise

Cardiofitness is a direct measure of a physical capability of the heart and its cardiovascular system. This includes its capability to deliver oxygen as needed. The heart and its related system involves substantial muscle. The capability of this muscle develops from exercise just as does the capability of any other body muscle. Muscles in arm, leg, and heart include those of differing types called slow twitch and fast twitch. As training proceeds, muscle cells, and especially the fast twitch ones, increase in size, usually over a span of 8 to 10 weeks.

There are training options for arm and leg muscles – within limits – of using lower weights and more repetitions or higher weights and fewer repetitions. But the primary factor that produces strength is exercise stress, or intensity, as produced for example by the size in pounds or kilograms of a weight lifted. Substantial intensity and a periodic increasing of this intensity make up the key to development of body strength. Muscle develops from exercise intensity, not from energy calories. For example, if we lift a 50-pound weight ten times and a 20-pound weight 10 times, we do not become capable of lifting a 70-pound weight ten times. The added strength improvement for also lifting the 20-pound weight may be negligible. It is mostly the highest intensity or the lifting the 50-pound weight that produces muscle.

The heart uniquely exercises itself. But the same principles of muscle development must still apply, as they do from resistance training. The heart can exercise only by beating faster than usual. The stress against heart and cardiovascular system muscle from the increased blood flow simulates the stress on the arm muscle produced from lifting a weight in resistance exercise.

As this stress builds cardio system muscle, the larger blood flow provides improved nourishment to the entire system of cells contacted by blood. This larger blood flow opens up channels throughout the cardiovascular system to provide improved contact between blood and other body cells. As in resistance exercise, exercise intensity is the key to the development of both cardio muscle and more efficient cardiovascular circulation.

Chemical engineering explains that the resistance to turbulent flow of a fluid in a circular fixed pipe at conditions present in the larger vessels of the cardiovascular system increases as the square of blood velocity. Although conditions in the pulsating cardiovascular system differ, it seems likely that the energy required and stress placed on cardio system muscle should increase at a higher power of the increase in blood flow rate. The research described in Chapter 4 shows that cardiofitness may develop at about the 1.6 power of the increase in blood flow rate above resting blood flow rate. This explains in part why higher exercise heart rates produce cardiofitness more effectively than do lower heart rates. Higher heart rates develop more than just proportional increases in the energy that exercises the cardio system.

How Resistance Exercise Increases Muscle

Much research has been done on how resistance exercise produces muscle. It is interesting to explore what happens during resistance exercise. This can help us understand better how cardiofitness can develop from exercise of the cardiovascular system.

Exercise research on muscle development identifies 1 RM as the maximum weight an individual can lift just one time. Individuals usually can lift lesser weights a number of times called repetitions. For example, if this 1 RM is 100 pounds, an average user can lift 60% of this weight 16 times, 80% of this weight 8 repetitions, and 90% of this weight 4 repetitions. Exercise is often done with a weight of 75% of 1 RM at can be lifted about 10 repetitions.

A resistance exercise program usually involves increasing the weight amount by just a few percentages each week or after each two exercise sessions. The amount of exercise intensity or weight level is the primary determinant of improvement in strength.

A completed single exercise of lifting the desired number of repetitions of a target weight is called a set. An exercise session usually includes a number of different exercises, each done for 1 to 3 sets. Research shows that there is a limit to the amount of exercise done each week that can increase muscle strength.

A study of 77 subjects on upper-body strength showed that doing 2 or 3 sets of a specified exercise produced little or no gain in strength vs. just doing 1 set over a 10-week training period. Another study of lower-body strength found a 14.5% increase for just 1 set per exercise session vs. only a slightly higher 15.5% increase for those that did 3 sets of the exercise during each exercise session. This tells us that there are specific limits to the extent at which muscle can develop from exercise during a one-week period. Doing more than this produces little or no further benefit. There is no clear relationship between calories of exercise used and strength development. Large amounts of calories beyond the amount needed to produce maximum muscle will produce little further strength benefit.

A very large study of 1132 persons found that muscle gains were 2.2 pounds for those doing 2 sessions a week and only 2.5 pounds for those doing 3 sessions per week for 8 weeks. An even larger study of 2776 subjects found identical increases in muscle strength of 3.1 pounds for those doing 2 and 3 sessions per week for 10 weeks. This tells us again that there are limits to the rate at which muscle will develop. You cannot force muscle to develop faster by doing more than a given amount of exercise each week. Some smaller studies found that 3 sessions per week of strength training produced more benefits than did two sessions. This can depend on how much exercise is done in each session. But in terms of actual time of resistance-exercise stress, there appears to be a limit to the amount of exercise that can be effective.

The finding that more than two hours a week of cardio exercise produces no further benefit in cardiofitness now becomes understandable. This two hours approximate the amount of exercise that can improve cardio muscle. More exercise than this at a given intensity is unproductive and largely wasteful of time.

The time limit for stress in improving other body muscles from resistance exercise may be much shorter than two hours per week. A set of body exercise can be done in only about one minute. Just one set done twice each week seemed to produce close to the maximum strength increase of a given muscle group for a given exercise weight. This involves much less time than the two hours of useful actual exercise stress per week for aerobic exercise.

The heart operates in a much different environment of exercise repetitions and amount of exercise load than occurs in the resistance training of large body muscles. It also is a pulsating system rather than a fixed muscle system. But the possibility exists that the limiting time for exercise effectiveness may by shorter at high intensities and longer at very low intensities than this two hours found for usual cardio exercise of the heart. Stress on muscle in weightlifting is an order of magnitude higher than the stress developed by increased blood flow in the cardio system.

This research and experience in resistance exercise explain why energy calories of exercise can have little or no effect in improving either muscle strength or cardiofitness. Exercise intensity is the key factor that produces muscle strength from each type of exercise. You probably could exercise hours every day with a small weight and burn large amounts of calories without improving strength very much. Similarly you could walk around the house periodically during most of every day and burn thousands of calories a week and not become very cardiofit. Increasing muscle requires a useful intensity of exercise.

There are other similarities in the way cardiofitness and strength from resistance exercise develop. Each develops most effectively over a period a 10-20 weeks. Each declines similarly after exercise stops. Each tends to reach a plateau level if some level of contributing exercise is maintained without change. This similar behavior supports further the fact that the improving of cardiofitness and the improving of other body muscle strength seem to be produced by similar processes of muscle building.

How Does Cardiofitness Produce Benefits to Health?

We next come back to that puzzle of how muscle development in the cardio system assists the widely differing biochemical processes that are involved in reducing risks of diseases. A likely answer is this: Cardiofitness is a highly selective marker of the effective higher than usual blood flows being developed throughout the cardio system.

First, coronary arteries can be pushed and kept much more open by the higher blood flow from cardio-type exercise. This widening of key vessels can substantially reduce risk of artery blockage. (See again the striking pictures in Figure 7-3 and other evidence in Chapter 7.) of the coronary artery diameters developed with and without cardio exercise.

These pictures demonstrate that the higher blood flows of regular exercise can substantially modify the physical structure of arteries. This specific enlargement of coronary arteries may be a reason why cardiofitness can have a larger effect in reducing risk of heart disease than it does in reducing risks of other diseases. Most ordinary physical activity that does not increase heart rate elevation sufficiently will not produce the regular periodic blood flow needed to accomplish and maintain this benefit.

Second, this same periodic increase in blood flow rate from cardio exercise will push thousands of miles of other blood vessels more open and improve chemical contact between nutrients in blood and cells throughout the entire cardiovascular system that reaches all parts of the body. This should enhance the benefits of nutrients in blood such as selenium and other antioxidants, minerals, vitamins, omega fats and other nutrients that can protect against heart and other diseases.

This larger distribution of blood nutrients in the body probably does not occur just during the higher blood flow rates during exercise. Rather, these higher flow rates of blood that produce cardiofitness also enlarge the vessels throughout the entire cardiovascular system similarly to way they enlarge coronary arteries. Cardio-effective exercise must be maintained at least periodically to keep these vessels more open and to retain these health benefits. If this exercise is not maintained, cardiofitness will gradually decline and blood vessel vitality will decrease.

Some Evidence Supporting This Scenario

We have multiple and confirming research on many nutrients in blood that shows that they can reduce risks of diseases via dose response. Specific results for how various diet and other nutrients in blood can reduce risks of multiple specific diseases are shown in many papers on the Life Ahead website (www.lifeahead.net).

There is other evidence supporting periodic increased blood produced by cardiofitness flow as a likely reason for the reductions in risk of disease. Other known potential causes explain only 20-25% of cardiofitness benefits for heart disease and only about 15% of overall cardiofitness health benefits on all diseases. This leaves 85% of health benefits not explained by any other known and verified causes. Improved distribution of nutrients in blood to body vessels could easily provide an explanation for most or all of this missing and principal cause.

Cardiofitness explains a substantial reduction in risk of coronary disease from its ability to widen coronary arteries. It seems clear that typical cardio type exercise can have a substantial effect on the physical state of cardiovascular vessels. Cardiofitness reduces risk of a large number of different diseases. It is unlikely that any single biochemical mechanism could explain these multiple reductions in risk. Improved contact with blood nutrients with other body cells could produce the differing biochemical processes required.

The finding that cancer is much better protected by cardiofitness than by ordinary physical activity suggests that increased blood flow rate is a primary factor involved in reducing risk. The key difference between cardiofitness and other forms of exercise is that cardiofitness selectively identifies higher than usual exercise intensities.

The surprising finding that most or all types of cancer are protected similarly by a given change in cardiofitness points to a common mechanism at least for this group of diseases. Improved contact between nutrients in blood and cells throughout the body could explain this similar effect on all causes of cancer.

The Heart Theory of Exercise and Cardiofitness

The fact that exercise benefits are produced best by exercise at the higher than usual heart rates that best improves the cardiovascular system has long been widely recognized. The Heart Theory contributes some new concepts that have not been adequately recognized.

227

1. The benefit of exercise develops from the same type of muscle building that strengthens arms and legs. Muscle building proceeds at a limiting rate. Thus there is a limit to the amount of exercise done in a given time period that can be useful in muscle improvement..

2. Exercise intensity is a primary need to develop muscle building in both resistance type exercise and in aerobic exercise of the cardiovascular system.

3. There is a limiting duration of exercise that can be effective in the development cardiofitness and other body muscle at any given intensity. This limiting duration in aerobic exercise is about two hours of exercise per week.

4. The exercise intensity of the cardiovascular system is improved by the rate of blood flow above that needed at rest maintained for useful time. The added energy of this increased blood flow improves the capability of the cardio system to distribute nutrients throughout the body. This added blood flow is a product of the increase in heart rate above that at rest and amount of blood included in each added heart stroke.

Note that maximum heart plays no role in this mechanism except to define a limit to the rate at which the heart will beat. Exercise heart rate comprises only part of the total increase in blood flow. Blood flow must also recognize both resting heart rate and amount of blood pumped per stroke.

The Heart Theory Explains Previous Puzzling Findings

The new theory explains all of the puzzling findings noted at the start of this appendix. It explains why energy calories can have either some effect or little or no effect in improving cardiofitness. It explains logically why there can and even should be a limit to the amount of exercise that is useful each week. It is two hours per week of highest intensity that counts. This is all the exercise that cardio muscle can absorb and process. This actual limit may vary somewhat with intensity of exercise.

The Heart Theory explains why benefits of exercise move up slowly mostly during a time of about 24 weeks of continued cardiofitness-type exercise. It explains why these benefits tend to plateau after most benefit is obtained, and decline slowly as exercise is stopped.

The Heart Theory also explains why large numbers of low-intensity exercise calories can produce only moderate benefits, and why much shorter times of more intense exercise calories can produce higher benefits. It explains why exercise intensity can be so much more important to the development of cardiofitness than is an equal calorie amount of exercise duration. This better circulation of blood nutrients also could explain the improvements in serum cholesterol also develop from cardiofitness.

A Verification of the Heart Theory

Chapter 3 described how a planned experiment developed cardiofitness from two groups that exercised at the same amount of energy calories but at differing levels of exercise intensity. Those exercising at the higher intensity obtained much larger improvements in cardiofitness.

The Heart Theory forecasts this result quantitatively with reasonable accuracy. The Master Table forecast that the group exercising at the higher heart rate and exercise intensity should at same calorie amount produce an advantage of 12 in CFR. The actual difference measured was 14 in CFR. These are substantial differences in cardiofitness produced by equal numbers of exercise calories.

As noted and referenced before, three other research projects found the same result. Increasing exercise intensity at the same measured calorie total produced a substantial further improvement in cardiofitness. These results are uniquely explained by the new Heart Theory. The calorie theory again fails these tests completely.

A Modified Heart Theory

The present Heart Theory holds that cardiofitness from usual aerobic-type exercise develops from the highest intensity maintained for about two hours per week. A broader form of the theory could be that the maximum effective time of exercise depends in part on exercise intensity. The effective time of more intensive resistance exercise could be shorter, and the effective time of low-level exercise at heart rate elevations below 30 beats per minute could be longer than this 2 hours per week. Our present evidence is limited to exercise time per week. It is also possible that there is a daily limit to the amount of exercise that is useful for improving cardiofitness. I prefer this modified theory but could find no adequate evidence to support it.

We do have epidemiological evidence that the benefits of occupational physical activity add to that from aerobic leisure time physical activity. In its present pure form the Heart Theory would forecast no benefit for adding exercise at a lower intensity to that from two hours or more of exercise at some higher intensity level. The Modified Theory might be able to explain how large amounts of lower-level physical activity, such as that in some occupations, could produce some useful benefits and supplement gains from aerobic-type exercise. Another possibility is simply that higher amounts of occupational physical activity also on average produced higher actual heart rates for the minimum time each week.

The new Heart Theory opens up many new ideas for physiologists to study. Does good aerobic exercise add as much to the cardiofitness of persons in active occupations as it does to those in inactive occupations? Does an hour of exercise at lower intensity plus 2 hours at higher intensity produce a higher cardiofitness than just the 2 hours at the higher level? Suppose we add 3 hours at the lower level to the 2 hours at the higher level. Will this now produce a difference in cardiofitness? Results from experiments like these could suggest an improved form of the Heart Theory of Exercise and Cardiofitness.

APPENDIX 6

How to Use the Life Ahead Program for Exercise and Cardiofitness

The Life Ahead computer program, a free computer download, can identify your likely levels of cardiofitness and physical activity calories from any kind, intensity and duration of exercises. The program can compute your cardiofitness level from a wide variety of exercise tests. And it also can indicate your risk of major diseases and your healthy days of life ahead for any exercise or combination of exercises. It can approximate the results of the Master Tables of cardiofitness from entries of exercise heart rate for different exercises.

Download and Start the Program

Go to www.lifeahead.net and click on option to download the Life Ahead program. Start the program from the screen icon, or if this not found, from lifeahead3.exe in the program folder location C:/program files/life ahead3. The opening screen as the left image following should display.

First try the demo program by clicking it from startup display. Read the information as noted in the right image, enter your age and click Continue to show the Start Up display. The program includes help for all displays and should be easy to use without going through the procedure that follows. But I will outline it for those interested.

Click on the User Name for your gender, and click the upper button for Enter or Edit Wellness Information. You do not enter a name into the demo program in the next screen shown, but complete the other items asked for as gender, height, weight, smoking habits, exposure to smoke and pollution, and general type of physical activity you do other than exercise. You do not enter Optional Items

Press Continue when these entries are finished. You will then bring the important and powerful Entry of User Exercise and Estimate of Cardiofitness display. This is shown in larger format following:

Figure AP6-1

Exercise Entry Form in The Life Ahead Program

The Exercise Entries

The entries that show in the demo program are typical US population values. You can enter hours per week and an estimate of intensity of any combination of different exercise groups such as walking, jogging or running, other aerobic exercise, weight, calisthenics, or resistance training or sports. Alternately, you can enter a usual exercise heart rate when performing any of the first four of these exercises. If you have an average heart rate for sports, enter this as Other Aerobic. You must have entered a Low Resting Heart Rate for the exercise heart rate options to operate.

Values at lower right show estimated gains in cardiofitness in CFR for doing the last-entered exercise and the maximum gain from any entered exercise. Cardiofitness as per the Heart Method will develop from the maximum intensity maintained of any individual exercise entered. A starting value of CFR is estimated from the selection of your Physical activity without Exercise in the previous entry screen. The value at lower center for CFR represents a sum of this starting CFR and the CFR from the exercise entered in this display.

You should experiment by entering values for different exercises to learn how this display develops all results instantly as entries are completed. Keep in mind that cardiofitness does not develop from a sum of values from different exercises. Only the higher intensity of exercise achieved for two hours each week contributes to cardiofitness.

The present program will compute aerobic exercise results only for the exercise that develops the highest fitness. If you do two or more different aerobic exercises with the most active one done for less than two hours per week, there will be some contribution from a second exercise. For this result, enter only the exercise done most intensively, and enter the total time for both or all exercises in the time or duration entry of this exercise. Do not enter results for more than one exercise unless only a physical activity calorie result is desired.

Calories of exercise are also shown at the lower right. A starting value for exercise calories per day is estimated from your Physical Activity Other Than Exercise in the previous display. Calories per day from the last entered exercise and from a total of starting calories and all other exercises entered are shown at the Totals display. Unlike the estimates for cardiofitness, which are based on highest intensity of exercise, calories are developed from a total of different exercises entered. Calories computed are the more correct net values rather than the misleading and higher total values often cited.

Values for maximum heart rate are based on 90% of the most accurate formula as shown in Appendix 4. These heart rates will be useful only for those that are accustomed to vigorous exercise

Try Computing a Result

On completion of a useful exercise entry, you can Go Back to Start to the Name Selection and startup display then compute results for an average population. Select the Compute Results option, ask for an average diet and press Continue twice to go through diet displays that should not be changed for a demo result.

Figure AP6-2

Main Results from the Life Ahead Program

% RISKS of MAJOR DISEASE of a POPULATION of AGE 50 HAVING AVERAGE RISKS and HABITS and GOOD HEALTH HABITS with DEMO WEEKLY DIET No 1				
DURING 10 YEARS to AGE 60 FOR MEN of AGE 50				
	AVERAGE HEALTH RISKS		RISKS at GOOD HABITS	
HEALTH CAUSE	% Disease	% Death	% Disease	% Death
Heart Disease	9.9	3.1	0.6	0.2
Stroke	1.6	0.4	0.2	low
Cancer,All Causes	8.6	3.4	4.6	1.3

Basic Risks and Habits provide a likely 9120 Future Well-Days (25.0 Yrs) of Healthful Days from Age 50.

Good Habits might provide 4900 Future Well-Days or 13.3 More Yrs of Healthful Life

-- Explore Risks vs. Different Habits --

Diabetes			
Colon etc. Cancer	Change Ages for Above Risk Estimates	Change Other Factors	Health Value a Food
Prostate Cancer		Weight	Value Vs Other Diet
Lung Cancer		Exercise/Fitness	Value Another Diet
Heart Diseases	Macular Degeneration	Get More Well-Days!	Value Supplements
Help Info	Dementia, Alzheimer		
More Help Info	List All Diseases	Diet Analysis	Return to Start Menu

The Main Results display will show extensive results for this entry, as in Figure AP6-2. This includes estimated future healthy days and how many more might be achieved by better health habits. The risk of heart disease and cancer is shown for a next ten years. Please read the Help Info to learn how the program will compute the benefit of almost any possible change in exercise or other habits. The results from the demo program will be for an average US population for the entered age and exercise.

The Get More Days option shows estimates of the habits that can be improved and the amount of Well-Days potential for improving each habit The extensive Diet Analysis shows how diet can be improved. Any results from the demo program will be for a typical US population for the entered age and other factors.

Compute Results for a Change in Exercise

To learn how a change of exercise can change outlook for risk of disease and Well-Days of life, click on the Exercise/Fitness option under Change other Factors to take you back to the exercise entry screen. Try an entry of more or less exercise, and click Compute Results. This will bring up a new computation showing the differences in risk of disease and in Well-Days ahead for the different exercises versus the results of your previous entry. You must go back to the Start menu and press Reset to start a new reference entry.

Estimate Your Own Cardiofitness Ratio, or CFR

Life Ahead provides an extensive range of options for estimating or computing your actual cardiofitness level in CFR. You access these options by clicking the Enter Fitness Measure option in the above Entry of User Exercise display. This display follows:

Figure AP6-3

Cardiofitness Tests and the CFR from the Life Ahead Program

You MUST Click CALCULATE button at right following completion of each test entry to compute a result.

	Test Used	Heart rate at 3 minutes	CALCULATE
From a Specific Treadmill Test	⊙ Test A No Incline. 3.5 mph		
	○ Test B 2% Incline, 3.5 mph		Reset Entries
	○ Test C 5% Incline, 3.3 mph		

From a Bicyle Test
Heart Rate at 3 Minutes

From the Bruce Method

Highest Level Attained	Minutes Into Last Level	VO2 Max Measured by any method

Your Cardiovascular Fitness in CFR:
   90 is poor; 100 average; 115 good; 130 excellent

Treadmill Basis	From Bicycle	Bruce	VO2 Max
Exercise 98.3		Avg Other Tests	

Back to Exercise	Info: Life Ahead Fitness Tests	Return to Start	Continue

235

The upper entries ask for treadmill tests A, B, or C, as described in Appendix 2 or in the program Info. You enter your heart rate after three minutes into the test. You MUST press the Calculate button to develop a result from any test entry. A CFR value from a treadmill entry will show at lower left opposite Treadmill Basis. You also will note a value opposite Exercise that represents a value of CFR estimated from the exercise you entered.

Your actual cardiofitness may vary from the average due to genetic and other reasons. You also can enter cardiofitness results from an exercise bicycle exercise test, the Bruce Treadmill Method, and from an actual measured entry of VO2 Max. Each result will be shown separately in the lower output display. The values from different tests probably will vary somewhat as each measures different functions of the body, and each measurement involves some margin of error. Thus it is best to use just one method in tracking your progress in improving cardiofitness.

The Treadmill test basis is taken as a most usual reference, and this basis when available will be used for the Actual CFR. Alternately, if a treadmill test is not entered, the program will compute and use an average from all other entered measurements. Again, a comparison of CFR values for a given individual must be made from the same test or test combination.

Treadmill Test C should be a useful and simple test if you have exercised regularly. Results for Tests A and B are computed values that are not fully tested and are for those that are not now in very good physical condition. An adjustment for resting heart rate is not now available. Such an adjustment could improve accuracy of the test. It is hoped that researchers will do more research on these cardiofitness tests that are practical for people to use.

Using the Life Ahead Program

Life Ahead is a powerful program for producing wellness from a very large variety of other lifestyle actions. Although its demo program will produce useful results for most people, more pertinent and accurate results can be obtained by entering more about your own habits and risks. Restart the program from the opening display or ask to Start a New User Name from an opening display. Press Continue after finishing your exercise entries then enter your habits and factors. Ask your doctor's assistant for one or two cholesterol and blood pressure values if you do not have them. But you can enter these later if you wish. The program will use average population values for any entries you do not make. Please read much more about the program in the program information displays.

Life Ahead provides the most comprehensive entry and scientific valuation of diet now available. Much more about the program is included in the program help and in papers on the Life Ahead site. The benefits of your exercise can somewhat depending on your diet and other lifestyle factors. Nearly a hundred mostly easy to read scientific papers are provided on the Life Ahead site, which describe and verify the health factors included in the Life Ahead program. Many of these papers include uniquely the actual results of all or most useful research studies published

APPENDIX 7

Impressive Research Confirms the Value of Cardiofitness

Some of the extensive evidence showing that cardiofitness is far more important to health and longevity than usually estimated from exercise was shown in Chapters 1 and 7. But there is much more evidence about the benefits of cardiofitness that is now quantified as the CFR. To keep readers from becoming bogged down with all this evidence, I brought some of it back to this Appendix section. This should be of interest to researchers, analysts and those interested in scientific evidence.

The idea that cardiofitness was the probable factor that reduced risk of heart disease was widely accepted even prior to 1970 by physiologists and other experts. This was the basis for the exercise then proposed to the public. I describe here first, the results of my 1980 Global Scientific Analysis and its subsequent confirmation from research in following years. Second, I show results of a statistical meta-analysis of much of the same research that uses an approach more familiar to those doing health research. Each analysis provides in quite different ways a convincing demonstration of the importance of cardiofitness.

1. A GLOBAL SCIENTIFIC ANALYSIS

Effects of Estimated and Actual Cardiofitness on Risk of Heart Disease and Death

My previous book provided what I believe was the first scientific confirmation that cardiofitness is the probable key factor that reduced risk of heart disease by exercise. I reviewed every useful published study the probable physical activity calories developed by study groups and the probable cardiofitness that would result from their exercise. About 50 research study comparisons had been published relating various measures of exercise to risks of heart disease. The results for the value of cardiofitness were striking and conclusive.

Figure AP7-1 is a reprint of the early study results in the Pulse Point Plan.[19] The only change is the name HPI for the measure of cardiofitness, which I now prefer to call the CFR. Consider first the top left plot for all coronary heart disease. Each little circle represents the risk of disease or death obtained in a research study for a higher cardiofitness group as a percentage of the risk of lower cardiofitness group. The values are plotted at their estimated difference in cardiofitness in CFR as is shown along the bottom scale. Each point represents information from a complete research study of different groups. By definition the points must pass through the origin at zero effect for zero difference in CFR. As the CFR or cardiofitness difference between groups researched moves higher, the risk of all coronary disease moves lower. The higher is the CFR of an exercising group, the lower their risk of coronary heart disease.

The trend noted for coronary heart disease in the top left chart is repeated similarly for other groups that suffered myocardial infarction (heart attacks) at the top right, and for other groups that suffered death from coronary disease at bottom left. The chart at lower right shows that risks of death from all causes on still other groups also were related to differences in CFR.

No actual cardiofitness measurements of CFR were then available. All CFR values were estimated for the different populations based on the amount and kind of physical activity that was involved. The plots show a reduction in risk of each category of heart disease from 100% to about 20% for a CFR advantage of 22 or 22%. This means that those groups that exercised to a 22% higher level of cardiofitness developed only 1/5th the risk of

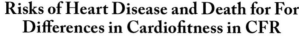

Figure AP7-1

Risks of Heart Disease and Death for For
Differences in Cardiofitness in CFR

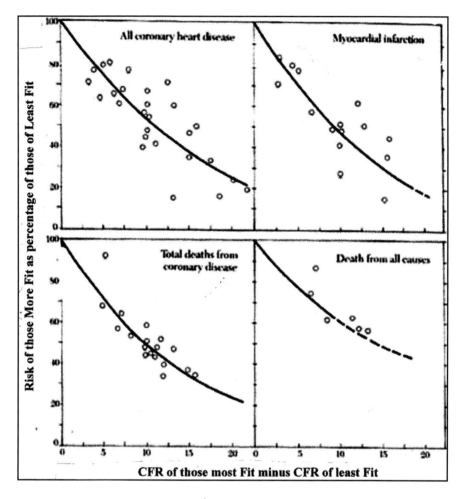

these different types of heart disease as did those that did no exercise. The risk of death from all causes from those that developed a similar difference in cardiofitness was about 2½ times lower for those the did not exercise.

The Global Analysis of research represented in Figure AP7-1 included all the useful research relating cardiofitness to heart disease and death found published before about 1980. Each little circle in this chart represents the results from an entire study, usually from results on several thousand individuals. The result from this forecast made during and before

1980 suggested that the risk of heart disease and death from all causes was related at highest significance to differences in cardiofitness.

Although not shown here, there was no useful relationship then between calories of physical activity and risk of heart disease. Highest benefits were associated with comparatively modest numbers of exercise calories involved in leisure time exercise. And highest likely calories of physically-active occupations produced only moderate changes in risk.

Confirmation from Measured Cardiofitness

Results started to become available from research that related risk of heart and other diseases to actually measured values of cardiofitness starting a bit later in the 1980's. The agreement with the new actual results with the earlier forecast results was excellent. Previous Table 1-1 in Chapter 1 showed that these results for cardiofitness dwarf the usual 1.5 to 2 times maximum benefits associated with other measures of physical activity.

Figure AP7-2 shows a powerful demonstration of the global importance of cardiofitness. The ordinate of this chart shows, as in AP7-1, the risk of the higher CFR group as a percentage of the risk of a lower CFR group. The abscissa shows the difference in CFR between these groups. Thus this chart shows how risk of cardiovascular disease diminishes as cardiofitness in CFR increases.

The open circles and black solid line show the values for risks of cardiovascular diseases vs. estimated values of the CFR as shown in above Figure AP7-1 for pre-1980 research that was published in my 1982 book. The solid circles are for results from studies published since 1983 based on actually measured values of CFR. These solid circles from more recent research show remarkably good agreement with my previously estimated effect of CFR on coronary death shown in Figure AP7-2. This is true for risks up to the maximum 20%-22% increase in CFR identified from the pre-1980 research. But the solid circle values that represent results from actually measured values of the CFR now extend to much higher differences in CFR. These results point to a 10 times reduction in risk of coronary heart disease death from higher improvements cardiofitness as CFR.

Figure AP7-2 represents an effect of cardiofitness on risk of disease from estimated and measured values of CFR from about 70 studies that include results on more than 2 million men and women. Again, each little circle represents result of an entire research study usually involving several thousands of people.

241

Figure AP7-2

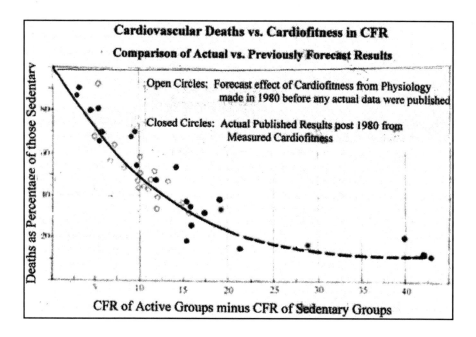

This confirms from two quite different methods that the primary causative agent in all studies probably was cardiofitness. The same results were obtained from exercise and physiology as were obtained later by actual measurement. A high goal of research is to forecast a result from a theory and have that result confirmed later by direct measurement. This was done directly for the measurable condition of cardiofitness and risk of heart disease.

In conclusion, we now have a more than a half-century of research showing that cardiofitness has a major effect on the risk of cardiovascular diseases and death from all causes. No such extensive confirmation of the importance of cardiofitness has to my knowledge been published elsewhere.

Cardiofitness Appears to be a Primary Causative Factor

A comparison extensively discussed by researchers has been 'physical activity vs. physical fitness.' These have commonly been viewed as are two separate, different and even competitive factors. The results in Figures AP7-1 and AP7-2 and the repeated failure of physical activity to produce a useful separate effect on risk of heart disease beyond that measured for cardiofitness suggest that the concept of 'physical activity' and risk of disease may be a non-item. Effects of other verified factors such as blood pressure, cholesterol and inflammation could account for any remaining effects identified as physical activity that are not accounted for by cardiofitness. Yet as discussed in Chapter 7, even these other verified factors also appear to be developed by the same exercise that produces cardiofitness.

It seems possible – and perhaps even likely – that all or nearly all risks shown as 'physical activity' from research probably identified results for amounts of cardiofitness present that simply were not measured.

2. A META-ANALYSIS[82]

The Global Scientific Analysis method that seeks to identify underlying basic causes of behavior is not usually used by health researchers. Results of health studies are presented as statistical ratios of a disease or other statistical results for persons having a different amount of some factor. These ratios of risk from individual studies usually have a substantial error margin. A meta-analysis combines the results of all or best studies published to develop an average risk and overall error margin of this average risk.

A usual meta-analysis of exercise – and at least one of these has been published – cites an average percent reduction in risk from exercise in all studies and its standard error. This analysis is virtually useless because it tells us nothing about what kind of or how much exercise produced this average result. It just assures us that something called "exercise" usually is good to do.

A more sophisticated and more informative than usual meta-analysis has been published, however, that provides a statistical comparison of what is now commonly called physical activity and physical fitness. I call this physical fitness measure more accurately as cardiofitness.

Physical activity refers to the activity of individuals separated into groups by answers to various questionnaires about their physical activity. Most of these questionnaires attempted to produce estimates of calories of physical activity expended. There usually is little useful correlation between measured cardiofitness and exercise calories from questionnaires of a given population. Most published research on exercise has been based only on these questionnaires about physical activity.

The Meta-Analysis of Interest

This 2001 study by Paul Williams of the Life Sciences Division of Lawrence Berkeley National Laboratory first compared the results of 16 general studies of this physical activity with results of 7 studies of measured cardiofitness. This study pooled results of included studies to obtain risks of cardiovascular disease per percentage of amounts of physical activity or physical fitness (or cardiofitness). The sixteen studies of general physical activity included results on 1,012,000 individuals and the studies of cardiofitness included 312,000 persons.

Figure AP7-3 shows that the groups that were measured by physical fitness or cardiofitness obtained a far greater reduction in risk of all cardiovascular diseases. The risk ratio of about 0.6 identified about a 40% reduction in risk of cardiovascular disease for the studies of general physical activity. The cardiofitness group moved toward a risk ratio of 0.3 that identified a 70% reduction in risk.

Figure AP7-3

- -

Risks of Cardiovascular Disease and Associations with Physical Activity and Physical Fitness

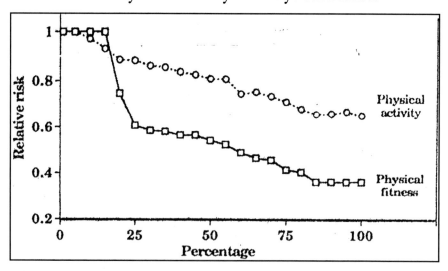

This first group of studies were those included in the Surgeon General's report of 1996. Williams then added further studies published since this report to a total of 30 studies of general physical activity and 8 studies of cardiofitness. This increased the population of individuals included to 2.6 million individuals. The result was a plot near identical to that of Figure AP7-3. The difference between results was significant to a probability of less the 0.0005.

The result for the cardiofitness group for results below 15% of total is puzzling. The researchers did not measure values in the first 10% level of cardiofitness. Thus I do not feel that this statistical discontinuity represents a real effect.

A key observation from this comparison is that cardiofitness develops an entirely different level of risk than do usual measures of physical activity. This is another comparison based on the very large body of available research. This quite comprehensive statistical confirmation provides a direct comparisons of risk that is independent of the CFR or any other method of assessing cardiofitness. Cardiofitness was measured at different levels by a variety of different exercise tests in the various research projects.

Although the Global Scientific method develops much larger potential effects of cardiofitness than the statistical method, I think this meta-analysis provides an important confirmation of the fact that cardiofitness measures a condition of the body that is an order of magnitude more important than that from other known estimates of physical activity.

The author states as conclusion that "Being unfit warrants consideration as a risk factor, distinct from (physical) inactivity and is worthy of screening and intervention." This is essentially a key conclusion of this book. As I have said elsewhere, this potentially major health risk for low levels of cardiofitness is now completely overlooked by our health establishment.

Cardiofitness May Explain All of the Results

A major difference between this statistical approach and the Global approach is that this statistical method produced only an average benefit for cardiofitness from 7 or 8 studies. The Global method shows that there are wide differences in the cardiofitness level in CFR of the different studies included in this average. This explains further the important contribution of cardiofitness to risk.

For example, the included Cooper Institute men and women had reductions in risk of cardiovascular disease of 87% and 89%, respectively. But the group obtained this from a very large exercise difference of about 50 in CFR. The included Copenhagen study of men, which was carried for an overlong 17 years and reached a reduction in risk of only 43%, had an estimated difference in CFR of only 15. The included US railroad study groups that were followed for a long 17 years showed a reduction in risk of only 34% and also obtained a low probable difference in CFR.[16]

Thus the lower plotted line in Figure A7-3 for physical fitness could be replaced by a fan of lines for different levels of CFR. The plot for the difference in CFR of 50 would extend down close to a risk of 0.1, or one tenth. The plot for a 15 difference in CFR would be above the present plotted line.

I noted further that there may be no such thing as an added casual effect of physical activity on disease beyond that from measured cardiofitness. All physical activity will produce cardiofitness to some extent. The studies that measured both differences in physical activity calories and cardiofitness found no separate effect for physical activity, and that the effect of cardiofitness was dominant.

Thus the single lower line in Figure A7-3 could be replaced by a fan of lines for differences in cardiofitness, or CFR. The upper line in Figure A7-3 theoretically could be represented by another fan of lines for different amounts of cardiofitness in the different studies that were not measured. These two fans of lines could merge to form just one fan for differences in cardiofitness that only were partly measured in most of the research we now have available. No added effect might remain for what is called physical activity.

Interestingly, if we start with a hypothesis that cardiofitness is the primary cause of disease risk differences from exercise, it would be very difficult today to show from objective analysis of available research that physical activity as measured by calories develops any further change in or contribution to this risk.

REFERENCES

1   Yarvote, P. M., Thomas J., et al "Organization and Evaluation of a Physical Fitness Program in Industry" J Occup Med 1974, 9:589-598.

2   Morris, J. N., Heady, J.A., et al "Coronary Heart Disease and the Physical Activity of Work" Lancet 1953, 265:1053-1057.

3   Morris J. N., Kagan, A., et al "Incidence and Prediction of Ischaemic Heart Disease in London Bus Men" Lancet 1953, 2:553-559.

4   Morris, J. N., Chave,S. P., et al "Vigorous Exercise in Leisure Time and the Incidence of Coronary Heart Disease" Lancet 1 1973 333-339.

5   Morris J. N., Clayton, D. G. et al "Exercise in Leisure Time: Coronary Attack and Death Rates" British Heart Journal 1990, 63:325-334.

6   Blair, S. N., Kohl, H. W., et al "Physical Fitness and All-Cause Mortality" JAMA 1989; 262-2401.

7   Arraiz, G. A., Wigle, D. T. and Yang Mao "Risk Assessment of Physical Activity and Physical Fitness in the Canada Follow-Up Study" J Clin Epidemiol 45:419-428.

8   Ekelund, L. G., Haskell, W. L. et al "Physical Fitness as a Predictor of Cardiovascular Mortality in Asymptomatic North American Men" N Engl J Med 1988; 319:379-84.

9   Sobolski, J., Kornitzer, M., et al "Protection Against Ischemic Heart Disease in the Belgian Physical Fitness Study: Physical Fitness Rather Than Physical Activity?" Am J Epidemiol 1987 125L 601-10.

10 Lie, H., Mundal, R., Erickssen, J. "Coronary Risk Factors and Incidence of Coronary Death in Relation to Physical Fitness. Seven-Year Follow-up Study of Middle-aged and Elderly Men"

11 Peter, R. K., Cady, L. D. et al "Physical Fitness and Subsequent Myocardial Infarction in Health Workers" JAMA 1983, 249:3032-56.

12 Hein, H. O., Suadicani, R., Gyntelberg, F. "Physical Fitness or Physical Activity as a Predictor of Ischaemic Heart Disease? A 17 Year Follow-up in the Copenhagen Male Study."

13 Sandvik, L., Erikssen, J., et al "Physical Fitness as a Predictor of Mortality Among Healthy Middle-aged Norwegian Men" N Engl J Med 1993, 328:533-7.

14 Lakka T. A., Venalainen J. M., et al "Relation of Leisure Time Physical Activity and Cardiorespiratory Fitness to the Risk of Acute Myocardial Infarction in Men" N Engl J Med 1994; 330:1549-54.

15 Mora, S., Redberg, R. F., et al "A 20 Year Follow-up of the Lipid Research Clinics Prevalence Study" JAMA 2003, 290:1600-07.

16 Blanding, F. H. "Cardiofitness and Risk of Cardiovascular Disease and Death from All Causes" http://www.lifeahead.net/hef-paper-cvd-risk.htm

17 Gulati, M., Pandey D. K. et al "Exercise Capacity and Risk of Death in Women. The St James Women Take Heart Project" Circulation 2003 108:1554-1559.

18 "Physical Activity and Health A Report of the Surgeon General. NIH Centers for Disease Control and Prevention, National Center for Chronic Disease Prevention and Health Promotion, 1996

19 Blanding, F. H. The Pulse Point Plan Random House New York 1982.

20 Blanding, F. H. "Walking and Cardiovascular Disease" http://www.lifeahead.net/walking-chd.htm.

21 Kahn, H. A. "The Relation ship of Reported Coronary Heart Disease Mortality to Physical Activity of Work" Am J Pub Health 1962, 53:1058-67.

22 LaCroix, A. Z., Leveille, S. G. "Does Walking Decrease the Risk of Cardiovascular Disease Hospitalizations and Death in Older Adults?" J Am Geriatr Soc 1996 44:113.

23 Hakim, A. A., Petrovitch, H. et al "Effects of walking on Mortality among Non-smoking Retired Men" N Eng J Med 1998, 338:94.

24 Manson, J. E., Hu F. B., et al "A Prospective Study of Walking as compared with Vigorous Exercise in the Prevention of Coronary

Heart Disease in Women." N Engl J Med 1999, 341:65.

25 Lee I. M., Rexrode, K. M. et al "Physical Activity and Coronary Heart Disease in Women: is 'No pain, No gain' Passé?" JAMA 2001, 285:1447.

26 Tanasescu M., Leitzmann, M. F., et al "Exercise Type and Intensity in relation to Coronary Heart Disease in Men" JAMA 2002;288:1994.

27 Manson, J. E., Greenland P., et al "Walking Compared with Vigorous Exercise for the Prevention of Cardiovascular Events in Women" N Engl J Med 2002, 347:716.

28 Noda H., Iso H., et al "Walking and Sports Participation and Mortality from Coronary Heart Disease and Stroke" J Am Coll Cardiol 2005; 46:1761.

29 Blanding, F. H. "Exercise and Cardiofitness" http://www.lifeahead. net/exerciseandcardiofitness.htm

30 O'Donovan, G., Owen, A., et al "Changes in Cardiorespiratory Fitness and Coronary Heart Disease Risk Factors After 24 Wk of Moderate or High Intensity Exercise of Equal Energy Cost" J Appl Physiol 2005, 98:1610-25.

31 Gossard, D., Haskell, W. L. et al "Effects of Low and High Intensity Home Based Exercise Training on Functional Capacity in Healthy Middle-Aged Men" Am J Cardiol 1986; 57:446-49.

32 Crouse, S. F., O'Brien, B. C. et al "Training Intensity, Blood Lipids and Apolipoproteins in Men with High Cholesterol" J Appl Physiol 1997, 82:270-77.

33 Kraus, W. E., Houmard, J. A., et al "Effects of the Amount and Intensity of Exercise on Plasma Lipoproteins" N Engl J Med 2002; 347:1483-92.

34 Ready, A. E., Naimark, B., et al "Influence of Walking Volume on Health Benefits in Women Post- menopause" Med Sci Sports Exerc 1996, 28:1097.

35 Naughton, J. P, H.K Hellerstein and I. C. Mohler, eds. Exercise Testing and Exercise Training in Coronary Heart Diseases Academic Press, New York 1971 p 129-16.

36 Moon, J. K. and Butte, N. F. "Combined Heart Rate and Activity

Improve Estimates of Oxygen Consumption and Carbon Dioxide Production Rates." J Appl Physiol 1996 81:1754-61.

37   Warrren, B. J., Nieman, D. C., et al "Cardiorespiratory Responses to Exercise Training in Septuagenarian Women" Int J Sports Med 1993, 14:60.

38   Zhang, J. G., Ohta, T., et al, "Effects of Daily Activity Recorded by Pedometer on Peak Oxygen Consumption (VO2peak), Ventilatory Threshold and Leg Extension Power in 30-69 Year Old Japanese without Exercise Habit" Eur J Appl Physiol (2003) 90:109-113.

39   Blanding, F. H. Step Counts, Cardiofitness and Health http://www.lifeahead.net/StepcountsCFR.htm

40   Kramsch, D. M., Aspen, A. J., et al "Reduction of Atherosclerosis by Moderate Conditioning Exercise in Monkeys on an Atherogenic Diet" N Eng J Med 305:1483-89.

41   Mitrani, Y., Karplus, H. and Brunner, D, "Coronary Atherosclerosis in Cases of Traumatic Death." Medicine and Sport, Vol 4: Physical Activity and Aging, edited by D. Brunner and E. Jokl, pp. 241-48: Baltimore University Park Press, 1970.

42   Mann, G. V., Spoerry, A. et al "Atherosclerosis in the Masai" Am J Epidemiol 1972, 95:26-37.

43   Mann, GV, Shafer, R. D., and Rich, A. "Physical Fitness and Immunity to Heart Disease in Masai" Lancet 1965, 2:1308-10.

44   Church T. S., Barlow C. E., et al "Associations between Cardiorespiratory Fitness and C-reactive Protein in Men" A Arterioscler ThromB Vasc

45   Dufaux B., Order U., "C-reactive Protein Serum Concentrations in Well-trained Athletes" Int J Sports Med 1984, 5:102-106.

46   Blanding, F. H. "Diabetes" http://www.lifeahead.net/diabetes.htm

47   Wei, M., Gibbons, L. W. et al "Low Cardiorespiratory Fitness and Physical Inactivity as Predictors of Mortality in Men with Type 2 Diabetes" Ann Intern Med 2000,132:605.

49   Blanding, F. H. "Alzheimers Disease and Dementia" htpp://www.lifeahead.net/dementia.htm

50   Blanding, F. H. "Respiratory Diseases (COPD)" http://www.lifea-

head.net/respiratorydisease.htm

51 Blanding, F. H. "Macular Degeneration" htpp://www.lifeahead.net/macular.htm

52 Klein, R., Klein, B. E., et al "The Association of Cardiovascular Disease with the Long-term Incidence of Age-related Maculopathy: The Beaver Dam Eye Study. Ophthalmology 2003, 110:1273.

53 Blanding, F. H. "Osteoporosis" http://www.lifeahead.net/osteoporosis.htm

54 Blanding, F. H. "Arthritis and Health Risk" http://www.lifeahead.net/arthritis.htm

55 Blanding, F. H. "Life Ahead, its Basis and Method" http://www.lifeaheaadbasisandmethod.htm

56 Blanding, F. H. "The Life Ahead Program" http://www.lifeahead.net

57 Neaton, J. D., Wentworth, D. "Serum Cholesterol, Blood pressure, Cigarette Smoking, and Death from Coronary Heart Disease: Overall Findings and Differences by Age for 316,099 White Men. Multiple Risk Factor Intervention Trial Research Group Arch Intern Med 1992, 152:56.

58 Blanding, F. H. "Smoking, Cancer, and Cardiovascular Disease" http://www.lifeahead.net/smoking.htm

59 Blanding, F. H. "Blood Pressure and Cardiovascular Disease" http://www.lifeahead.net/bloodpressure.htm

60 Blanding, F. H. "The CFR- A Useful Measure of Physical Fitness" http://www.lifeahead.net/HEF-paper.htm

61 Robinson, S. "Experimental Studies of Physical Fitness in Relation to Age" Arbeitsphysiol 1938, 10:251-323.

62 Allard, C. "Commentary, Physical Activity and Cardiovascular Health" Can Med Ass J 1967, 96:879-81.

63 Gyntelberg, Finn "Physical Fitness and Coronary Heart Disease in Copenhagen Males aged 40-59 II" Danish Med Bull 1973, 20:105-11.

64 Stofan, J. R., DiPietro, L. "Physical Activity Patterns associated with Cardiorespiratory Fitness and Reduced Mortality: the Aerobics Center Longitudinal Study" Am J Public Health 1998, 88:1807-13.

65 Passmore, R. and Durnin, J. V. "Human Energy Expenditure"

Psychological Review 1955, 35:101-140.

66　Braith, R. W. and Steward, K. J. "Resistance Exercise Training, Its Role in the Prevention of Cardiovascular Disease" Circulation 2006; 113:2642-50.

67　Tanasescu, M., Leitzmann, M. F. and Eric B. Rimm, "Exercise Type and Intensity in Relation to Coronary Heart Disease in Men" JAMA 2002; 288:1994-2000.

68　Blanding, F. H. "Concepts Differ in Biochemical Engineering Analysis; Multiple Regression, to often an Invalid Method" http://www.lifeahead.net/concepts-biochemical-eng.htm

69　Takeshima, N. Rogers, M. E. et al "Effect of Concurrent Aerobic and Resistance Circuit Exercise Training on Fitness in Older Adults" Eur J Appl Physiol 2004;93:173-182.

70　Len, C. Lai, J. S. et al, "12 -Month Tai Chi Training in the Elderly: Its Effect on Health Fitness" Med Sci Sports Exer 1998 30(3):345-51.

71　Fradkin, A. J., Gabbe, B. J., Cameron, P. A. "Does Warming up Prevent Injury in Sport? The Evidence from Randomised Controlled Trials?" J Sci Med Sport 2006 Jun (3):214-20.

72　Thompson P. D., Funk, E. J., et al "Incidence of Death during Jogging in Rhode Island from 1975 through 1980" JAMA 1982 247:2535-38.

73　Hu, F. B., Stampfer, M. J. et al "Physical Activity and Risk for Cardiovascular Events in Diabetic Women" Ann Intern Med 2001 134:96-105.

74　Rockhill, B., Willett, W. C. et al "Physical Activity and Mortality: A Prospective Study among Women" Am J Public Health 2001,91:578.

75　Naughon, J. P., H. K. Hellerstein and I. C. Mahler eds. Exercise Testing and Exercise Training in Coronary Heart Diseases Academic Press, New York 1971, p. 129.

76　Hagberg, J. M. Graves, J. E. et al "Cardiovascular Responses of 70-79 yr-old Men and Women to Exercise Training" J Appl Physiol 1989 66:2589-94.

77　Broeder, C. E., Burrhus, K. A. et al "The Effects of Either High-intensity Resistance or Endurance Training on Resting Metabolic Rate Am J Clin Nutr 1992, 55:802-10.

78   Huang, G. Gibson, C. A. et al "Controlled Endurance Exercise Training and VO2 Max Changes in Older Adults: A Meta-analysis" Prev Cardiol 2005 8:217-222.

79   Blanding, F. H. "Exercise, Cardiofitness, and Cardiovascular Disease" http://www.lifeahead.net/exercise-fitness-cvd.htm

80   Blanding, F. H. "Exercise and Cardiofitness – A Summary" http://www.lifeahead.net/exercise-Fitness summary.htm

81   O'brien, B. J., Wlibsko, J. et al "The Effects of Interval-Exercise Duration and Intensity on Oxygen Consumption during Treadmill Running" Sci Med Sport 2007, 29:290.

82   Williams, Paul T. "Physical Fitness and Activity as Separate Heart Disease Risk Factors: A Meta-analysis" Med Sci Sports Exerc 2001 33:754-756.

83   Haskell, W. L., Lee, I-Min, et al "Physical Activity and Public Health: Updated